Through the Rabbit Hole
navigating the maze of providing care

The Comfort in their Journey Series
by Trish Laub

A Most Meaningful Life
my dad and Alzheimer's
a guide to living with dementia

Peaceful Endings
guiding the walk to the end of life and beyond
steps to take before and after

Through the Rabbit Hole
navigating the maze of providing care
a quick guide to care options and decisions

Through the Rabbit Hole
navigating the maze of providing care

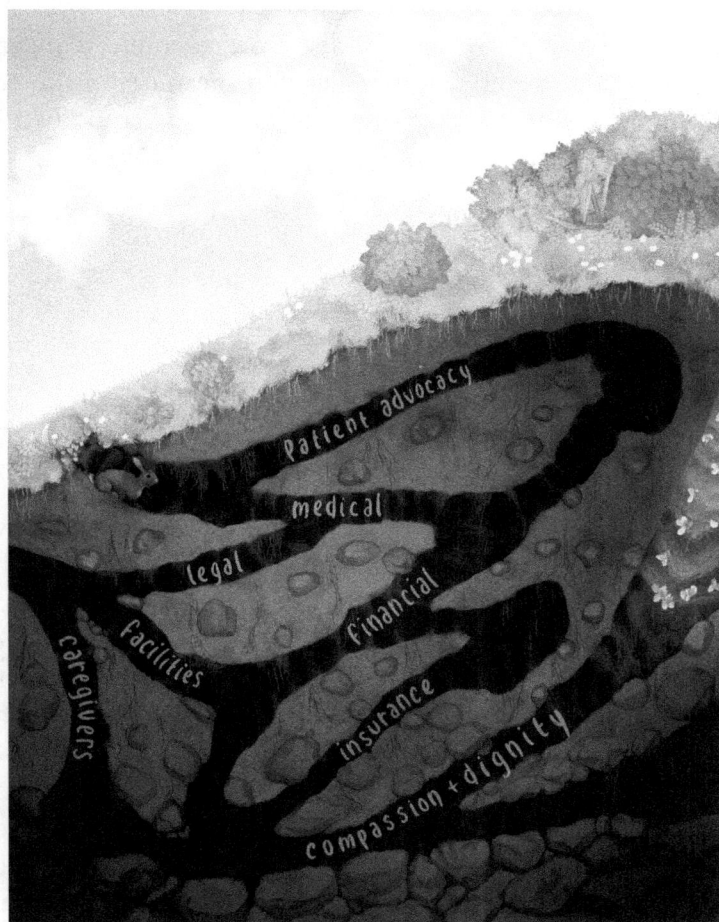

a quick guide to care options and decisions

Trish Laub

PSM Publishing

Through the Rabbit Hole … navigating the maze of providing care   by Trish Laub

Cover Illustration: Laura Tharp
Author photo: Joanne Wagner
Published by: PSM Publishing

ISBN-13: 978-1-7322006-2-3
Library of Congress Control Number: 2018939961
First Edition   Printed in the United States of America

PsM
ublishing

To purchase:
www.TrishLaub.com   303-900-2845
6845 Osprey Ct Highlands Ranch CO 80130

Dedication

To my mom
I need your grace to find my own.

ACKNOWLEDGEMENTS

with special thanks to both Mom and Dad,

my husband, Chris, who supported my absence during this experience as well as the creation of this project,

my sisters, Barbara and Nancy, who lived my experience with me yet have their own experiences and stories to share,

my daughter Justine, who is my inspiration for all things,

the friends (Janice, Karen, Skye, Julia, Mia, Teilene and others) who have carried me through the dark times,

those who have encouraged me to shine a light down the path for those who come next,

Roseanne Geisel (editor), Joanne Wagner (author photographer), Krista Lee (logo and graphic designer), and Sophia Taylor (website/branding) all of whose excellence is unsurpassed,

Deb Sheppard, medium and mentor, who helped me with the "Great Clearing," making this project possible,

all of the caregivers who loved my parents and taught me so much: *Margery, Debbie, Lucia, Ann, Ruth, Shawn, David* and *Angel,* as well as many others who provided not only care but unconditionally gave love; they are all extraordinary people and I am proud to know them and to call them family,

and especially, all of the exceptional professionals who provided care for our parents, in particular *Joe Omdaio RN,* who set the bar for outstanding nursing care; *Mike Zdero OT,* who not only taught my sisters and me how to safely maneuver our parents but also how to motivate our dad; *Dr. Karen Wendel,* infectious disease specialist, who still possesses the curiosity that drives her excellence; *Dr. Kenneth Blake*, colorectal surgeon, who saw our mom as a vibrant 90-year-old woman worth treating; and *Dr. Charles Nutting*, interventional and diagnostic radiologist, who reminded us that there is something much greater than our individual abilities that determines the outcome of the journey,

and finally a very special thank you to all those who agreed to be what I call my "small book" readers, those who read and provided invaluable feedback on the content: *Justine, Janice, Karen, Skye, Cathe, Margery, Ellen, Judy, Elisabeth, Susie, Klaralee, Debbie and Chris.*

CONTENTS

Chapter 10
SENIOR CARE ...

Chapter 11
HELPFUL DURABLE EQUIPMENT
NONDURABLE EQUIPMENT
AND SUPPLIES ...

Chapter 12
DEALING WITH SPECIFIC MEDICAL ISSUES ...

Chapter 13
FINAL THOUGHTS ...

POSTSCRIPT ...

OTHER RESOURCES

NOTES TO THE READER

Citation of Information

This book presents a conceptual understanding of information, terms, and statistics intended to assist you in a conversation with, and in asking questions of, a professional. Information, unless specifically cited, was provided to me during conversations with professionals or through research of many reliable sources. I have tried to simplify it for non-professionals.

Patient Advocacy

Patient advocacy is **the most important role** in regard to caring for another, and can literally be the difference between life and death. The topic is mentioned in every book of the Comfort in Their Journey book series. It is discussed in Chapters 6 and 11 of *A Most Meaningful Life* and Chapter 1 of *Peaceful Endings*. However, if you only read one chapter in the entire series, please read **The Need for Patient Advocacy... the most important role,** Chapter 2 in *"Through The Rabbit Hole."*

Pronouns

At some point in your life, it is almost certain that you will be responsible for the care of another person. It may be a parent, a sibling, a child or a friend. It may be a loved one, and it may be someone for whom you do not feel love. The gender and age will vary. These variables make it difficult when writing a book and having to reference the person for whom you are responsible for providing care. Therefore, in this text, in regard to the gender, the pronoun "their," as a genderless person, may be used.

About the Ladybugs

The ladybug has been an obsession for me since I was very young and began to collect them. My dad named his fishing boats Ladybug and Ladybug II. The use of the ladybug is an homage to my dad, and the red color, my mom's favorite and her most recent nail color, an homage to her.

Comfort in their J🐞urney
with *Trish Laub*

You may notice that the *Comfort in Their Journey* logo incorporates the ladybug as the "o" in the word journey.

The open-winged ladybug appears at the top of special sections, such as the Dedication and the start of the Contents, and on the page prior to the start of each chapter.

The closed-winged ladybug appears at the start of each subchapter. In addition, while all information in the book is important, the presence of 🐞🐞 two closed-winged ladybugs is used to indicate information that requires additional attention. The presence of 🐞🐞🐞 three closed-winged ladybugs indicates especially critical information.

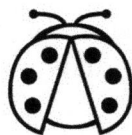

Knowledge is Power.

PREFACE ...
an unlikely expert ...
and "short is the new black"

I became an unlikely "expert"; it's as simple as that. I am not a medical, legal or financial professional. My expertise is derived from the full-time care of my parents, one with Alzheimer's, for whom I delivered the total care and the end-of-life experience that my parents desired.

In the book "Outliers," the author Malcolm Gladwell speaks to what truly makes someone reach their potential for success. He shares that more than IQ, and in addition to many other factors, practice is key to becoming successful. The principle states that 10,000 hours of "practice" or experience that pushes the skill set to the brink are needed to achieve mastery in any field.

Recently there was an ad for Denver's UCHealth in which Peyton Manning says: "It takes 10,000 hours to become an expert at something. But what happens at 20,000 hours? Or 30,000 hours? What happens when you dedicate yourself to it? Do you become something greater? A leader? A mentor? An innovator? At a certain point, it seems, you stop playing the game and start changing it."

My experience puts me well over 12,000 hours of "practice." Does it make me an expert? Maybe, but only on what I experienced. And after experiencing what I have, it might have seemed "easy" to just walk away and never talk about it or share what I have learned with anyone. To simply "move on." But, I couldn't do it -- walk away with all that I have learned and experienced. It became a "calling," the desire to share in hopes that it might help even one other person thrive in a situation which many times offers only frustration and often defeat. A calling, but was I an expert? Yes, and I am qualified.

What am I qualified to offer? I offer my story and my experience. It is highly likely that during your lifetime you will be responsible for the care of a person with a severe health issue and equally as likely that it will be during the final years and days of that person's life. I offer you the opportunity to *thrive* throughout the process, to think and then take action.

I am here to offer you information, some direction and suggested questions to ask.
- I am not a medical professional; I am not providing medical advice.
- I am not a legal professional; I am not providing legal advice.
- I am not a financial professional; I am not providing financial advice.

During my experience, I needed information I didn't know how to find, and I needed it quickly. Since my experience, I have found that there are hundreds of books and organizations offering pieces of the information I needed. And while the Internet offers information, extreme caution and verification are necessary to ensure accurate and useful advice. In many cases I didn't even know where to look for it or the terminology to Google or to ask. In other cases, I had too little time to find, read and understand it all. I needed the Reader's Digest version of everything. I needed a guide: a clear, concise and useable quick reference. With that in mind, I have adopted the philosophy that "short is the new black" – it is not the volume of words but the value of them that is useful; that providing you with lists and bullet points, things to consider, questions to ask and leads to follow are the most helpful delivery of information.

I also want to state up front that many factors, ranging from geographic proximity to financial resources to flexibility of work schedules, determine what is possible for every family or caregiving team. Each family or caregiving team will handle things in a way suitable for them and the person relying on them. My hope is to provide you tips and spark ideas that work for you.

In short, I became an unlikely expert; I have lived what I have to share.

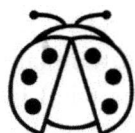

Dearly beloved,
We are gathered here today
to get through this thing called life.
Prince

PROLOGUE ...
"how did we get here?" and the resultant crisis

With the exception of one or two necessary procedures in their lifetimes, my ancestors, including my parents, were very healthy. When my parents' health went into crisis, each parent at the age of 90, I found myself standing amid a world about which I knew nothing. "How did we, our culture, get here?", to a place of specialists and facilities such as assisted living, skilled nursing, skilled rehabilitation, memory care and nursing homes. My maternal grandparents had been cared for in my parents' home, with the exception of my grandmother being hospitalized for a few days for additional comfort care at the end of her life. I now found myself in a world where a majority of elders are spending more time in emergency rooms, hospitals and other facilities, each with its own requirements and offerings, as opposed to being cared for at home or in the home of a family member. The health care system is a world I did not understand but suddenly had to navigate.

The Practice of Medicine
To answer my question, I began to read a lot about the practice of medicine from ancient times to the present. I found quite an evolution. In just a few millennia we have progressed from a time when the workings of the internal body and the existence of germs were unknown, when a simple cut could lead to infection and death and medical instruments or medications were limited or scarce. Here are some of the most interesting facts that I learned:

1

- The **first medical school in the United States** was created in 1765. (University of Pennsylvania University Archives and Records' University History, School of Medicine: A Brief History.)
- In 1847, the **American Medical Association (AMA) was created** to provide standards for medical education. (Encyclopedia Britannica.)
- Without many tools, the doctor's function was often to provide comfort to his patients.
- It wasn't until 1900 that things began to change rapidly. In 1910, only a little over a century ago, there were **155 medical and osteopathic educational institutions** in the United States and Canada granting doctoral degrees. But 89 of those institutions quickly closed due to substandard education and no minimum admission requirements. (Loyola University Stritch School of Medicine: The History of Medical Education.)
- After World War I, several important events took place. In the 1920s, **modern surgery and the use of groundbreaking treatments to control contagious diseases with reliable prescription drug**s became options. Both penicillin and insulin were discovered. (Encyclopedia.com)
- In 1928 **medical residencies** were created to allow for a training experience post education.
- As chemistry and physics advanced, so did medical education. The **first successful organ transplantation** was performed in 1954. (Stanford University history archives.)
- Now, in the 21st century, the use of **surgical lasers and robots, high-powered magnetic imagers and the advertisement of pharmaceutical drugs** directly to the patient are commonplace.

The Medical Providers

Even the role of the medical provider has rapidly evolved. U.S. Baby Boomers' experience with a family doctor was an occasional visit to a private office. Often even babies were delivered at home. In my lifetime, family doctors had office hours during which you would "walk in" without an appointment, sign your name on a piece of paper and be seen in the order of arrival. If an issue was serious, a family doctor would visit the patient at their home. In the rare event that a patient was hospitalized, the family doctor would oversee their care and visit the patient in the hospital.

By the time I was providing care for my parents, the medical care model had changed to include a variety of medical providers. Family doctors, now called Primary Care Providers (PCP), often no longer provide inpatient care, which instead is turned over to a hospitalist employed by the hospital to oversee care and to send updates to the PCP. A PCP most often is an internal medicine specialist, who refers their patients to other specialists when necessary. New medical specialties continue to arise, such as the relatively recent creation of palliative and hospice care. The specialization has continued to develop with the creation of Physician Assistants and Advanced Practice Registered Nurses, which include four specializations requiring additional education.

The Care Facilities

Next, I wanted to understand the creation of care facilities: why they exist, what they are and what they offer. Following are the key events I found in the evolution of facilities:

- In the "old" days, as people aged they were moved into a family member's home to finish out their days. Sometimes an aging family member exhibited signs of being "crazy," or senile, but they were cared for and kept safe without the need for a specific label. There were few diagnoses, let alone pharmaceutical options for relief of symptoms for what we now label dementia or Alzheimer's, nor for other serious illnesses such as cancer. With few alternatives, people were provided with dignified care, delivered with compassion and comfort in a family environment.
- Several historic events, such as the U.S. industrial revolution and the Civil War, made it impossible for many families to care for their elderly, incapacitated and/or destitute relatives. **Almshouses** were created to care for those whose family members could not provide care, including orphans. It was a far less than desirable solution.
- In the 20th century, charitable organizations began to establish **private homes for specific needs** resulting in the almshouses consisting almost entirely of the elderly poor. The problems with almshouses prompted several government policies and regulations in an attempt to abolish them during the 20th century. It became clear that there had to be a separation of those who required personal nursing or medical attention and those who required only financial support. The nursing home industry was created with a great deal of government involvement.
- By the 1950s, policymakers were successful at **abolishing almshouses and allowed for the development of public and private institutions** for the neediest older adults. In addition, after WWII many families moved from their place of origin in search of work, making it difficult to

later provide care for those elders who had not moved with the family. The demand for nursing homes became too great and not without problems.

- By the 1980s, **nursing homes** began to take the shape with which we are familiar: preadmission screening to prevent inappropriate entrance and rehabilitation services.
- In the 1990s, **assisted living facilities** began to emerge providing care in a residential setting.
- The 21st century began with the further segmentation of the industry. This included **separation of nursing homes and stand-alone rehabilitation facilities and the prevalence of assisted living and senior communities**.

While this information is greatly oversimplified and summarized, it serves to explain the creation and rise of nursing homes and other care facilities.

The Crisis of Care

In 2030, there will be twice the number of persons 65+ in the country as there were in 2000. According to the Centers for Disease Control and Prevention, the number of persons residing in nursing homes by 2030 will double. There will be a 300% increase in the number of those over 85. Today there are approximately 44 million Americans providing care for an adult in need. The projection for 2030 is staggering.

What does all of this mean? It means that things have gotten complicated, and that we are headed for a crisis if the current care model doesn't change. I have an acquaintance in the elder care industry who says that even if we build all day, every day, we cannot build enough spaces for all those who may need care as they approach end of life. And as life expectancies continue to lengthen, it is not likely that the situation will improve. We cannot continue to depend on the government to fund our final days or on others to provide care during those days. Yes, we will likely need some assistance, but we need to understand the alternatives. We need to understand the terminology -- the lexicon of care. We need to understand the care system and take responsibility for our own care and that of our loved ones, in order to do as much as possible to stay well and independent of facilities.

We are on the horizon of a universal care crisis, and we have a collective responsibility to care for ourselves and our aging population. In 1900, life expectancy was 47 years: in 2017 it was nearly 80 years. As disease rates increase, the age of those needing care is decreasing. The need for care has grown rapidly.

What can we do about it? My solution is to stay as healthy and independent as possible for as long as possible. We no longer live in a time when we don't know the health risks of many consumables and lifestyle choices. And, knowledge truly is power. Out of necessity for my parents' care, I had to educate myself on how to navigate the care system and to understand the care options and necessary decisions. I have had to learn to be a patient advocate for those whose care I oversaw. And finally, in preparation for any care needs, I might have in the future, I have created and continue to review my estate and financial planning. (See Chapter 2 and the Afterword of *Peaceful Endings*.) I don't know what will happen in regard to care for me, but I will be as informed and prepared as possible to care for myself and to make caring for me as easy as possible for someone else. With my plan in place, I can move on with this thing called life.

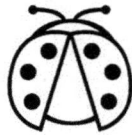

The light at the end of the tunnel
is not an illusion.
The tunnel is.
Unknown

INTRODUCTION ...
into the rabbit hole

In the spring of 2012, my family was unexpectedly thrown headlong into the world of health care. What was to have been a five-day skilled nursing rehabilitation stay for my dad turned into a nine-week nightmare and the beginning of a 2 ½ year journey of care for my parents. My family was totally unprepared to navigate the workings and nuances of medical care, Medicare and a variety of insurances, facilities, agencies, care providers and caregiver options, among other issues. I realized that, while the dimensions of Alzheimer's disease may have exacerbated our situation, our experience was universal and was what anyone with the responsibility for overseeing and/or providing care for another person would ultimately face.

As described in the Prologue, the medical and caregiving approaches that I knew as a young child have evolved, and for the good that the changes may have brought, with them have come extreme challenges. It has become complicated, and the days of blindly relying on your medical provider and the care system are gone. With so many moving parts in the system and medical issues involving a variety of specialists, it is easy to get lost. You can find yourself with no one acting as quarterback, coordinating information and determining the next play, and no one coaching the care team to success. The greatest need in regard to medical treatment and care is patient advocacy. You either have to accept responsibility for advocating for yourself or empower another to do it if you are unable. We live in a fast-paced, sound bite world full of too much information, much of which we do not even understand, and when it is part of the medical system, understanding it can mean the difference between life and death.

Through the Rabbit Hole is the story detailing my family's experience with traveling the maze that is care today, and includes the information and tools to facilitate that journey. It starts with the initial experience of falling into the unknown darkness of the rabbit hole where everything was unfamiliar, and where I found myself surrounded by a labyrinth of care components (medical, legal, financial, insurance, facilities, caregivers, patient advocacy, dignified and compassionate care) about which I knew little or nothing, and which required specific terminology I did not understand. It was the beginning of the odyssey of learning what was necessary about each branch of the maze and then navigating the options and decisions that would bring me to the light at the end of the tunnel.

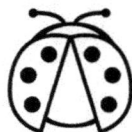

You either get bitter or you get better.
It's that simple.
You either take
what you have been dealt
and allow it to make you a better person,
or you allow it to tear you down.
The choice does not belong to fate
it belongs to you.
Josh Shipp

Chapter 1

A NEW RESPONSBILITY ...
managing care

In the introduction I said that seemingly overnight I was faced with the responsibility of providing care for my dad, who had Alzheimer's, and shortly thereafter also for my mom. It was my **choice**, which made all the difference. I never felt that I put my life on hold, but rather that I chose a new normal for my life. While what happened during those 2 ½ years was challenging, it didn't happen *to* me, it happened *through* me. It was an opportunity for me to rise to the challenge: to put into practice what I believe most and to show who I am at my core.

> It's during the worst storms of your life
> that you will get to see the true colors
> of the people who say they care about you.
> Unknown

The Choice to Manage Care
You have likely been asked to be responsible for the care of another. You may have planned on this day and are looking forward to the responsibility, or you may not have anticipated the request or feel that you are not cut out for it. Know that you have a choice; you are not required to do it. At minimum you are responsible for seeing that someone oversees the care. And, even if you decide that you can do it, managing someone's care does not necessarily mean providing the actual daily care.

What's Your Ability?

In the video "How to Live the Life You Never Imagined," disability rights advocate and speaker Richard Pimentel talks about the lesson he learned while in Vietnam when he was assigned a potential suicide mission. He says that responsibility is not something someone puts on you or a requirement of you, but rather your response to an ability. Do you have the ability to manage care, or provide care, or provide support to those who do? What will your response to that ability be?

There are many considerations in determining what level of responsibility you can assume: logistics such as proximity to the person, work commitments, family dynamics, finances, etc. All things considered, all you can ever do is to do the right thing for both you and the person who has requested your ability.

However, don't confuse a real lack of ability or willingness to respond positively to an ability with making excuses to take the easy way out of the situation. Few things in life worth doing are easy.

> Integrity –
> the choice between
> what's convenient and what's right.
> Tony Dungy

The Challenges You May Face

There are many challenges that you may face if you accept the responsibility to manage care for another.

First, assuming the responsibility for the care of another **does not** make you *durable power of attorney for health care decisions*. (See Chapter 2 of *Peaceful Endings*.) If the person requiring care management is capable of decision-making, a power of attorney is unnecessary. It is still prudent to identify who will have responsibilities in the future. Until then, the person needing care can make their care decisions. It may be wise to discuss the fact that designating the same person to manage care and to be medical power of attorney will simplify future care decisions.

While there are many obvious challenges in managing the care of another, the most important challenge is ensuring dignified and compassionate care. This is particularly difficult when managing care for an elder in a country that does not revere them. Working with a variety of caregivers, I was enlightened by the reverence of elders by those from other countries. As I explain throughout this book, the changing business model for medical care has become more difficult to navigate, especially for elders, and now often requires patient advocacy. (See Chapter 2.)

All in all, it requires a great deal of time and effort, combined with diplomacy in protecting the dignity of another. If your situation involves caring for a family member, there may be more challenges in store.

Sound stressful? Overwhelming? I have faced all of it and am here to help you navigate through the maze that is care today.

If you find yourself in a position to manage care from a distance, you may face additional challenges. You can do the following:

- Ask family and friends to assist with oversight, to be your eyes and ears.
- Centralize all information so that it is accessible by you and those who are local to the person in need of care.
- Consider whether a medical alert or personal emergency response system device would be helpful.
- Look into other technology that might make long-distance monitoring easier.
- If possible group medical appointments at a time when you can be present. If you cannot be present, you can call someone who will be present and listen in on the appointment.
- Look into local resources for assistance, such as for meals, transportation and for household and personal chores.
- Contact a senior center in the area where care is needed.

Crisis Management

This chapter covers several aspects of the crisis that can occur when you are faced with the responsibility of caring for another. This topic is covered in more detail in Chapter 1 of *Peaceful Endings*.

> Life has many ways of testing a person's will,
> either by having nothing happen at all or
> by having everything happen all at once.
> Paulo Coelho

The Importance of Having a Plan
Once the decision has been made to manage care, it is important to develop a care philosophy, goal and strategy for reaching the goal with the patient. (For a specific example, see *A Most Meaningful Life*.) This will allow everyone involved with the care to have a clear understanding of the patient's wishes, and a plan to deliver them.

As manager of the overall care, it is also important to have an understanding of the patient's estate and end-of-life planning. (See Chapter 2 of *Peaceful Endings*.)

Expect the Unexpected
Expect the unexpected in every situation, from being shortsighted due to a diagnosis to falling into the cracks between medical specialties. Just when you think you know what is going on, know that sometimes you just can't guess what will happen. You can spend hours and days trying to imagine every possibility and when you least expect it, something you never could have imagined will happen. And, with the unexpected outcome comes the rollercoaster ride.

My friend thought that her husband, who was battling cancer, was headed for hospice care as it was assumed that his ongoing symptoms were caused by the progression of cancer. We talked about every combination of events that we could imagine, most resulting in the end of life. After spending four days in the hospital, it was determined that the cause of his symptoms had nothing to do with his cancer and that he was not headed into his final days. Just when she thought that she knew what was going on, she was surprised both by the medical outcome and the emotional rollercoaster ride that followed.

Caregiver Stress

About a year into providing care for my parents, my sisters and I held a caregiver team meeting, which included seven nonfamily caregivers. Our concern was that we, my sisters and I, were beginning to get rundown and worried that we would eventually become ill due to stress. The research and statistics on family caregiver stress resulting in serious illness is substantial. The next day I saw a video in which it was stated that the negative impact of caregiving was directly related to perspective. Those who *chose* to provide care suffered far fewer negative effects from the experience than those who felt *required* to provide the care. I immediately knew that I would be fine, as it was completely my choice to care for my parents. Remember that whether you're caregiving or doing anything else, you always have a choice! (See Chapter 9 for more information.)

Self-Care... What is YOUR Medicine?

The one requiring care, especially if there is a diagnosis, is often given medication and possibly offered complementary treatments, such as massage, to help them feel better and heal. It is equally important that you receive care and maintain your wellness in order to be of the greatest help to another. Self-care is not self-ish, it is essential to your ability to be resilient. 🐞🐞🐞 Resilience is not how you merely survive, but how you recharge and thrive.

> Sometimes you just have to fluff your tutu,
> adjust your tiara, turn up the volume,
> and dance it off.
> Unknown

For me, my medicine is teaching and taking The Nia Technique mindful movement classes. They are mind-body based and the overall objective of the class is to feel better physically, mentally and or emotionally. The classes are based on the technique of nine movement modalities (martial, dance, and healing arts) structured into 52 moves. The movement works with eclectic music to quite literally shift things in the mind, body and emotions. My participation, whether as teacher or student, demands my complete awareness and focus, and removes me from the daily world while I work on making myself feel better. It is while doing Nia that I find peace.

Peace.
It does not mean to be in a place
where there is no noise,
trouble or hard work.
It means to be in the midst
of those things
and still be calm in your heart.
Unknown

What is your medicine? What do you do to feel better? What brings you peace? It may be meditation, reading, practicing yoga, taking a walk with a pet, honing some skill or talent, learning a new skill or anything that speaks to your spirit. For one friend, her medicine was what she called "Freedom Fridays." Friday was the day of the week that she "forgot" about her husband's diagnosis, didn't say the big "C" word (cancer) and pretended that he was well. Find your medicine, know it, use it. (See Chapter 1, *Self-Care is a Four-Letter Word; It is Self … LOVE!* of *Peaceful Endings* for more ideas.)

A critical part of self-care is building a care team that can over time relieve you, if only providing respite, from some of the areas of responsibility. (See Chapter 7, *The Support Team.*)

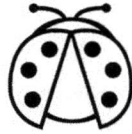

Literally the difference
between life and death.

Chapter 2

THE NEED FOR PATIENT ADVOCACY ...
the most important role

We all know that medical providers save millions of lives each year. Furthermore, we depend on these providers to keep us well, to repair what is broken, to replace what is worn out or to eradicate what is making us sick. I have seen medical professionals go way beyond healing, repairing and replacing and straight to what appear to be miracles. I have seen a person's quality of life improved immeasurably though surgeries the likes of which, seemingly from a sci-fi movie, I cannot begin to comprehend.

That said, there is a truth that requires our attention. Medical providers, on whom we depend particularly in life-threatening situations, have jobs that are difficult and sometimes require life and death decisions under extreme pressure. Those who work in critical or ongoing care are often responsible for too many patients at one time. In addition, medical providers now find themselves in a fast-paced, quickly changing environment. They face a constant stream of new information amid increasing constraints and difficulties from the health care business model. No matter how skilled the medical provider and how many medical and technological advances we celebrate, medical providers will always be human. The same humanity that allows for creative problem solving and innovation leaves room for error.

In May of 2016, a study by researchers at Johns Hopkins Medicine stated that medical error was the third leading cause of death, after heart disease and cancer, accounting for a projected 250,000 deaths per year. Other research done at that time projected that number to be as high as 400,000 deaths per year. That is potentially 1,000 people per day. Let that sink in for a minute! Although unacceptable, that number is somewhat understandable and realistically not totally preventable. While there may be no perfect solution, there is something that can help protect you and your loved ones and greatly reduce that number: patient advocacy!

While errors in the medical services are the greatest concern, patients and their families also can be hurt by financial errors related to the care. Medical claims must be filed with insurance companies and always require oversight and coordination, as does payment for uncovered expenses. The entire process is based on legal requirements and specifications with which a patient or family may not be familiar.

In all your roles in providing care, that of patient advocate is the most important. Again, you do not have to be the one providing the patient advocacy, but you then have to find another to do it. This chapter is long, as *it is the most important chapter in the <u>entire</u> book series.*

What is a Patient Advocate?

A patient advocate is a person who acts as the quarterback of a care team, coordinating and ensuring dignified and compassionate care and protecting the rights of a person in need of care. A patient advocate can be a family member or a professional. Professional patient advocates have a variety of backgrounds, from former clinicians to people who worked in the corporate aspect of health care or health insurance to those with life experience navigating the health care system. Some advocates will have earned the new national Board Certified Patient Advocate (BCPA) credential developed by the Patient Advocate Certification Board. The first round of certification exams was given in March 2018, and 149 advocates were certified. One way to find a professional patient advocate is to search the AdvoConnection Directory (www.advoconnection.com), which lists members of the Alliance of Professional Health Advocates.

The Need for Patient Advocacy

In the 2½ years I was managing my parents' care, I worked with many providers: medical, legal, insurance, etc. Some providers were outstanding, true rock stars in their fields. To those, I wrote personal letters of thanks. Some providers were not good to work with for a variety of reasons, and were "fired," resulting in the pursuit of one of the rock stars in their field.

In *A Most Meaningful Life,* I detailed my family's experience with the need for patient advocacy on behalf of my dad, who had Alzheimer's. It is a true story of our medical and care facility experience and sadly all too familiar. Here I am sharing my family's experience with the need for patient advocacy as we experienced during the care of my mom, which was similar but different to our experience with our dad.

This is *a brief summary of only one surgical/hospital experience, only one short example chosen from many others.* This series of incidences during one medical event occurred toward the end of the 2 ½ year care journey, when my family

23

was already familiar with the challenges of providing care, was prepared for what pitfalls lay ahead and was aggressively advocating for Mom. The hope is that by including it, you will have an idea of the many things that need oversight.

- We were sent by a medical provider to the emergency department (ED, previously called an emergency room or ER) to address two specific urgent concerns. When we arrived, the order for only one of the necessary consultations had been sent. **We waited 24 hours in the hospital for the necessary testing.**
- Mom's **medicines were entered into the system incorrectly eight times** before they were correct. We sat with a hospital employee each time the information was entered, and yet it would be incorrect the next time we checked the information.
- A hospitalist, whom we had never seen before, entered my mom's room and **announced a diagnosis before any testing had been done.** He based his *assumption* on her age and a previous, unrelated diagnosis. He said that surgery was not an option. A specialist arrived, disagreed, stated that surgery was an option and verified that the issue was in fact not related to the previous diagnosis.
- When surgery was required, **presurgical appointments were made for us**. Because we were also caring for our dad, the automated scheduling was never convenient or possible for our schedule, and it became a rescheduling nightmare. We should instead have been allowed to make our own appointments.
- We encountered an **enormous lack of communication** between the hospitalists and specialists. In addition to the already overwhelming workload for the RNs (registered nurses), they had to assume the responsibility

for being the hub of communication coordination.

- Mom had a chronic pain issue, one for which she would not do surgery because of her concern for my dad, that we had worked hard to keep under control with an approved non-narcotic pain medication dosage and a strict medication schedule. **The hospital pharmacy would not approve the dosage and discontinued the necessary prescription**. This contradicted my mom's protocol approved by her Primary Care Physician (PCP). The hospital's response was that mom was under the hospital's care and therefore its rules, regardless of whether it disrupted her previous care. This caused Mom to be in extreme unnecessary pain while in the hospital and upon her discharge it took us weeks to re-establish the protocol that relieved her pain.

- As part of mom's colostomy protocol, we gave her magnesium. Without giving it to her, we incurred several issues with her colostomy care. The hospitalist said they would not allow mom to take the magnesium because her electrolytes were good. The administration of magnesium had nothing to do with her electrolytes, but he could not understand the need based on her colostomy. Again, **we were told that mom was under the hospital's care and what her PCP and gastroenterologist instructed us to do was irrelevant**.

- After surgery, mom developed an infection and was moved to the ICU. We were told that there would be a family meeting to discuss the proposed care plan. Although we kept asking when we would speak with an ICU provider, there was no meeting. I walked into the room as the ICU RN was **going to administer an IV medication, to which my mom would have had a documented and potentially life-threatening adverse reaction**. No one was willing to speak with the family, and we were the keepers of the important information. Again, we were told that mom was under ICU care, however, the ICU provider didn't know mom's medical history.

- After mom left the ICU, there were several other issues. A certified nursing assistant (CNA) left the room to get something, leaving a tourniquet on mom's arm for more than 59 seconds, which is **a violation of protocol**.

- Physical therapy came to mom's room and when trying to get mom out of bed, caused her IV tube to get tangled in the IV tree, **causing mom's IV to be pulled out**.

- Most physicians would enter the room and not even look at mom. **They treated her like she was not even there**. Even if a physician looked at mom, they just saw an aging 90-year-old woman. A few physicians looked at her and saw the normally healthy and active woman who had a family that loved her, and who at the time happened to be really sick.

- **Discharge was always a challenge**, not just this time. Once we left the hospital, mom was no longer under the care of the hospitalist or specialists who had overseen her care there. In fact, if there was an issue after we got home, there was no one to call with a question or to ask for help, especially on weekends. When we tried to speak with someone at the hospital, we were told that they were no longer in charge of Mom's care and to contact her PCP. When we contacted her PCP's office, we were told to either make an appointment or to return to the ED. Many times this caused a cycle of recurring visits to the ED and admissions to the hospital, sometimes unnecessarily.

- Even when in-home health was ordered for Mom, there was **a lag between when hospital services ended and when in-home health services began**. It was never to be more than 24 hours, but often was.

- When we left the hospital after Mom's surgery, three antibiotics were prescribed, *each with a specific purpose and target infection*. **The hospital pharmacy would not fill all three prescriptions and sent us home with only two**. The third antibiotic, needed to prevent the suspected start of an infection in Mom's incision, was denied. A little over 24 hours later we were in the ED due to confirmation of the suspected infection. The infection, which could have been avoided with the third antibiotic prescription, created a wound that would take weeks of special wound care. Honestly, this event broke my mom's spirit, and she began to give up and decline after that.

- We were again home for a short time and had to return to the ED. After several attempts to get an IV into my mom's dehydrated, already painful and badly bruised arms, and after continuing to request that an ultrasound be used to find her vein or a Flight for Life member be consulted, **our request was finally begrudgingly honored.**

- We again were told that **Mom's pain protocol would not be approved**.

- When mom was to be released, for the third time in a month, which we felt was *again* too soon, I suggested that she might go to an LTACH (long term acute care hospital, see Chapter 6). **The doctors and nurses did not know what an LTACH was** and said that if I could arrange for it, they would sign the necessary paperwork.

- And finally, a word about test results. **The delivery and availability of the test results was inconsistent**. Often the results were available to me before the hospital staff had access to them and a few times they were never delivered to me.

Sometimes you have to
flip out and go bat s@$# crazy
to make a point.
Unknown

It is not my intention to just list off all the negatives. Again, it is to serve as examples of what can go wrong during medical care. With any negative, I want to be sure to identify the positive in our experience.

- The specialists, nursing staff and CNAs were attentive, responsive and appropriately confident.
- The RN/CNA to patient ratio was excellent, especially in hospitals with Magnet recognition, which made all the difference in their ability to provide quality care.
- Whenever possible, the RNs and CNAs cared for the same patients for several consecutive days. That continuity allowed them to get to know the patients and their histories, building patient confidence and comfort.
- RN rounding every hour was a productive and helpful practice.
- Access to electronic patient health records was helpful.

To this point, what I have provided has strictly been in regard to medical care in facilities. That is only one area in which patient advocacy is necessary. With each medical episode, there are resultant invoices and insurance payments. We had several instances in which invoices were incorrect and insurance payments inaccurate, requiring hours of time to resolve the discrepancies.

When my dad had surgery, we received the invoices, made insurance claims and paid the amount that was our responsibility. More than one year later, we received an

28

invoice from the surgeon's office for the services of a physician assistant who, unbeknownst to us, had been requested by the surgeon to participate in the surgery so that he could oversee the surgical follow-up. Medicare would not pay it as the PA was 1.) an additional provider that Medicare felt was unnecessary and 2.) the claim was filed past the one-year deadline. The surgeon's office wanted us to pay for the PA's services. We had never agreed to pay for anything additional, and it was the surgeon's decision to add him. We felt that the charges were not ours to pay. Therefore, we spent many hours working with Medicare to identify the details and timing of the claim and then working many more hours communicating with the surgeon's office. We ultimately did not pay for those services, but it required a family member to dedicate their time to resolving the issue. During a time of crisis, we might have assumed that we owed the money or it might have seemed easier to just pay the invoice instead of researching it.

Areas of Concern

Above I stated my experience with just one of my mom's medical episodes. During 2 ½ years of providing care for my parents, I experienced recurring issues. I bring attention to them so that you can be aware and avoid the pitfalls I experienced.

Although I provided pieces of the evolution of medical care in the Prologue, I want to summarize a piece of it again here. Doctors started largely by offering palliative care services, providing comfort in the absence of advanced tools and medications. Medical schools were later developed and taught specific protocols. Doctors were initially general practitioners, "jacks of all trades" who cared for entire families before the era of specialization. For decades the family doctor was your doctor during a hospital stay.

Today we have hospitalists and other specialists. We've all but eliminated the family practitioner, who was the physician most familiar with the patient and their history and could put them into the context of a family. Sometimes the PCP has been removed entirely from the hospital stay. Treatment only by specialists may result in not treating the whole person. Supposedly, they communicate with the other specialists, but my experience is that communication is failing miserably. The outpatient primary care doctors are struggling to stay in the loop through a volume of hospital reports.

The medical community provides an invaluable service, however, as with any large business – and **it is a business** – growth and rapid change have generated issues that need solutions.

Hospitalists

When I was growing up, it was rare to be an inpatient at a hospital, but if you were, your family doctor came to the hospital to oversee your care. This was good for the patient, as the doctor knew their medical history and provided continuity. In the late 1990s, the medical business model began to change in an attempt to improve the quality of care by employing doctors to be in residence at the hospital. By 1996 our family doctors (now called PCPs - primary care providers) no longer came to the hospital to care for us, and we began to hear the term hospitalist. A hospitalist is a doctor who provides medical care for hospital inpatients.

I understand the benefit for hospitals to employ or contract with hospitalists but while the business model may work for simple acute cases, the model did not work well for the critical and complex cases of my parents. During the course of a medical incident several hospitalists may rotate overseeing care. The situation is further complicated when a case requires the addition of one or more specialists, expanding the need for effective communication.

👓👓👓 Following are my experiences and my concerns.

- The hospitalists did not know my parents and never had an opportunity to develop a beneficial doctor-patient relationship with them. During several hospitalizations, my parents never had the same hospitalist more than a few days. Throughout a seven to 10-day hospital stay, over three shifts, we could easily see five or six different hospitalists. No hospitalist oversaw care for the entire hospital stay; care was constantly being turned over to the next hospitalist on duty.

  👓👓 This is not the fault of the hospitalists, it is a challenge of the medical care system business model.

- The hospitalists routinely overrode the protocols put into place by my parents' PCPs without understanding why that protocol was put in place. Upon return home, it would then take us weeks to get back to the protocols that had worked well for us before the hospitalization. This was a huge issue in regard to protocols for medications for Alzheimer's and pain.

- With rare exception, when one of my parents was hospitalized, the hospitalists did not seem to view them as an individual, but rather as just another patient. They generally did not speak directly to my parents and sometimes stated what they were or were not going to do without a diagnosis. Usually they only told us what

31

specialists would be consulted.

Of concern is the analysis of more than 560,000 Medicare admissions over the course of 2013, published in November 2017 by *JAMA Internal Medicine*. The result was that patients were 14% more likely to be discharged home, were 6% less likely to die within 30 days, and had 12% longer lengths of stay in the hospital when cared for by their PCP compared to those cared for by hospitalists. In addition, PCPs used consultations up to 3% more than hospitalists. The implication might be that the ongoing relationship and medical history the PCP has with the patient is of value in their treatment. But, it is not to say that being cared for by a hospitalist is a bad thing. For me, it says that there are holes in the business model, of which you need to be aware and provide advocacy for the patient.

Specialists
The move to specialization in medical practice continues to evolve with new areas being carved out. There are definitely benefits to specialization, but also challenges. The following is again my experience.

- Doctors are so specialized that no one is serving as a *holistic diagnostician*. The PCP used to be the diagnostician, but their role has been eliminated from the hospital stay. In theory, the hospitalist is to take on the role of the PCP during a hospital stay. However, *when a hospitalization is initiated by a specialist, they become the attending doctor* and a hospitalist is not involved.

- They are called specialists for a reason. They specialize in a very finite area of medicine. That works well until you have a problem that lies outside their area of expertise. Often additional specialists are brought into the care, requiring more communication.

Mom was in the hospital and doing well, until she wasn't. Every specialist came in the room and said that they didn't know why Mom was feeling so ill. The gastroenterologist and the infectious disease doctors said that Mom was healthy in regard to their specialties. The hospitalist had no ideas, as the specialists specific to Mom's case had cleared her. At the last moment, the infectious disease specialist said that she had a suspicion and decided to run a test that was not technically under her purview. She was correct, and Mom's illness was identified and treated.

Communication

- Having multiple hospitalists and/or specialists involved in a case necessitates communication among multiple departments. My experience was that because doctors in different departments usually didn't know each other, none of them really knew the care team members or the treatment plan.

- Communication among all the players was difficult and ineffective. RNs were the foundation of care and were left with the additional responsibility of trying to manage information and communication, often between multiple departments. I experienced an ongoing lack of coordination and communication.

- In 2012, a study conducted by Georgetown University projected that the United States would need 5.6 million more healthcare workers by 2020, an increase of more than 70 percent. The communication challenges are not likely to improve.

- Doctors must listen to the patient. While talking with a friend about her experience with caring for her parents, she said, "One of the biggest difficulties we had when my dad was sick was getting people to listen to what my folks wanted and needed. Everyone from the social worker to doctors all felt they knew best and made many assumptions about my parents and their resources that were wrong."

- Doctors must listen to the family. Most families are well intentioned and interested only in the quality and accuracy of the care of their family member. The family is the keeper of the patient's medical history. This is especially important with the variety of hospitalists and specialists who may have seen the patient over a period of time. Family members not only know the history of illnesses, but also the outcomes of medicines that the patient has been prescribed and other health-related considerations.

For example, any blood pressure reading taken digitally on my mom *would be incorrect*. For a correct reading, her blood pressure had to be taken manually using a stethoscope. Unless a family member was present when a blood pressure was taken, it was often taken incorrectly, potentially resulting in the prescription of unnecessary medication.

The Limbo Between Inpatient and Outpatient Care
- Upon discharge, the patient is left in limbo between inpatient hospitalist or specialist care and PCP care. The

minute you are discharged from the hospital, the hospitalist is no longer your doctor and is unavailable for questions; the specialists may be unavailable, and the PCP may not yet have the latest medical information. While you are instructed to schedule a PCP visit within a week of a hospitalization, it is sometimes difficult to get an appointment within a week and often the PCP has not caught up on your paperwork. If there are questions or concerns after returning home, in many cases the only recourse is to return to the ER.

We had a situation when, upon hospital discharge, oxygen had been ordered for my mom. While my mom was not even allowed to ride home in the ambulance without portable oxygen or before oxygen had been ordered for her home, we arrived home and hours later it still had not been delivered. It took me nine hours to get someone to respond to my call and to find someone who would address the situation. The hospital said they couldn't help me, because my mom had been discharged, yet a hospital employee had placed the order. Finally, arrangements were made to have the oxygen delivered in the middle of the night, 10 hours after discharge, during which time my mom had no supplemental oxygen.

- There was almost always a discrepancy regarding how we were to get care supplies upon discharge. The hospital would tell us that in-home health was to provide supplies, while in-home health told us that the hospital was to provide them. This caused us to scramble to locate and purchase our own supplies.

- Many times we were given prescriptions for medications. Sometimes our local pharmacy was closed by the time we would go to fill them. Other times the medications prescribed were not immediately available at our pharmacy. We found that while it was often more expensive to purchase the medications at the hospital pharmacy, it was easier and more effective.

The Teaching Hospital
Another consideration is the use of a teaching hospital. My mom was always open to being an inpatient at teaching facilities for three reasons. First, she understood that new medical providers need the opportunity to train with real patients. Secondly, she felt that teaching hospitals fostered the sharing of new ideas. Finally, Mom felt that it was good to have more people looking at her case.

There are several considerations.
- The patient often does not understand the role of each provider.
  - It is important to understand the hierarchy among the medical providers, as it allows for context on what is being said by whom and who has authority to execute orders.
  - The coming and going of many levels of medical providers can be confusing and a bit overwhelming. It causes the patient to continually repeat the same information to many people.
  - We literally created a flowchart of the participants in each department involved with mom's care. Sometimes medical providers would ask to see it in order to understand all the players involved in the case.

		PATIENT		
		patient name		patient support
		dignified/compassionate care		family/close friends
Date:	xx/xx/xx	**Attending Physician**		
Location:	*xxx hospital*	Specialty	*hospitalist, specialist*	
		Name		
		Fellows		
		Residents		
		Interns		

	Specialist	Specialist	Specialist	Specialist
Specialty				
Name				
Fellows				
Residents				
Interns				
Charge RNs				
RNs				
CNAs				
Phlebotomists				

- The hierarchy of providers means that they are always checking with their "superior," and ultimately their attending physician. The following is not a criticism, merely an observation and consideration.
  - Interns (generally called first-year residents now) and some residents in the earlier years of training do not have experience with the unusual. Residency allows them to gain that experience. When Mom's care was complex or critical, requiring experience and expertise, we were always sure that the attending physician was actively involved.
  - First-year residents are very much working from the standard protocols they have been taught. Residents in succeeding years have more experience. Fellows have completed their residencies and are doing additional training.
  - Across the United States, all residencies and

fellowships begin and end on July 7th every year. My mom had major surgery on July 1st and entered the ICU on July 2nd. Five days later, as she was being released from the ICU back to a regular unit, she found that all of the fellows and residents who had provided care for her were no longer there. She had an entirely new group of "trainees" who would ask all the same questions again and had to learn everything about her critical case.

- o Their hierarchy should not be our problem and in many cases it was.
- o There is a difference in the projection of "appropriate confidence" based on each person's level of experience. At times, it was a little like watching "peacocking," the ostentatious presentation of perceived worth. We had second-year residents that were overly confident and tried to speak above their perceived level of our understanding. On the other hand, we had attending physicians who could quickly evaluate without assumption or judgement the level of detail with which they could speak with us.

Protocols

It is true that medical schools teach protocols. If this situation happens, then you respond and treat that way. There are good reasons to have protocols. When protocols are learned, they can be used in high-pressure emergency situations with little thought. But relying purely on protocols, without considering individual, unique or extenuating circumstances, doesn't always provide the best option. Medicine is a science, but it is also an art.

My experience is that, while some medical providers continue to enjoy the hunt for the best solution for the individual patient, others have lost their curiosity, the thing that made them want to be a medical provider. Perhaps it is caused by burnout from overwork or frustration with the dictates of the current health care system.

> Instead of thinking outside of the box,
> get rid of the box.
> Deepok Chopra

Additionally, I found myself repeatedly asking, "Is this necessary or is this protocol?" Mom was in the ED and told that she needed an IV. It took three unsuccessful, extremely painful attempts to insert it, only to find out that it was not necessary for anything prior to the consultation and diagnostic testing that would occur the following day. It was protocol, but unwarranted in her case.

The Hippocratic Oath or Do No Harm
There is a misconception that medical providers "take" the Hippocratic Oath as part of their agreement to be a medical provider. Some do, others do not. It is an oath to adhere to a strict code of professional and personal conduct. That's a good thing. It is assumed that the phrase "do no harm" is part of that oath, yet it is not.

Until the past century, the interpretation of the phrase was fairly straightforward and a good thing. A medical provider did not take any action that could cause harm to the patient, and those actions were relatively clear. Yet with the advancement of medicine and technology, the context of the phrase results in new meaning. We have entered an era where, with good intention, lives can be extended through science and with technology to a time when quality of life no longer exists. What then is the definition of harm? It's something to think about.

> Whenever a doctor cannot do good,
> he must be kept from doing harm.
> Hippocrates

Another factor is that there are increasingly more options for treatment, some experimental. It is always the decision of the patient as to what lengths they are willing to risk quality of life for its extension. (See *Peaceful Endings,* Prologue.)

The Reality

For me, the overwhelming reality was that everyone (medical providers, RNs, CNAs, social workers) in the hospitals and facilities seemed to be aware of and share all of my concerns, but they all said that they didn't know how to get them resolved. The statement was that these are "administration problems," ones they were not in a position to change. They seemed almost defeated in the consciousness that big business had taken over, and they were helpless to effect positive change.

What to Do to Advocate for Your Patient

As I said previously, a patient advocate helps coordinate and ensure dignified and compassionate care and helps protect the rights and safety of a person in need of care. They also work to provide the patient or patient's family with the necessary, accurate information to make the best decisions in accord with their medical and legal wishes. The patient advocate then follows through to ensure those decisions have been communicated to all members of the health care team. *The medical care system and medical insurance are businesses.* There are many aspects of the system and often many people involved with each part. Medical providers are human and therefore susceptible to error. Everyone needs protection from big business and medical error.

Organization and communication are the key to patient advocacy. Knowing what the patient wants is critical to delivering the care that they desire. Many of the examples provided further in this book, regarding what we did in specific situations, are examples of patient advocacy. Following are some key aspects of patient advocacy.

Medical:
- Understand the diagnosis, treatment options, and the *questions to ask so that informed decisions can be made.* We gathered information, typed it up so that Mom had a copy to reread later, and went over it with her. We provided the information so that she could make her own decisions.
- Confirm a diagnosis – *second and third opinions.* When my Mom received a cancer diagnosis, she was seen by an oncologist at that hospital. Mom was then moved to another facility in which we requested a second opinion. We were told that the oncologist at the second facility could not evaluate Mom because she had been seen by another oncologist. That is not true. You have the right to be seen by other medical providers for second and third opinions.
- *Verify prescription name and dosage* and make sure they are administered correctly. We had daily log sheets which we used at home to ensure that medications were administered correctly. Whenever medications were given, the medication name and dosage was verified, and the person administering the medication then initialed the log.

- Understand the health care system and medical specialties involved with the patient's care. Flowchart the medical providers: PCP, specialists, multiple providers on the team within a specialty and those in training.
- Research diagnoses, medications, treatment options and providers.
- Facilitate shared decision-making with individuals.
- Assist patients in gaining comfort in communicating with and directing questions to medical providers.
- Coordinate care so all providers and care-team members have all information.
- Keep copies of all medical documents.
- Attend medical appointments when necessary.

Overall care:
- Chart the care team: know each team member, their name and their specific job and responsibility
- Document EVERYTHING, each meeting, each appointment and each conversation. Be specific, stating exactly who said what to whom. Document each medical episode in a different spiral notebook.
- Protect patient dignity: Ask yourself – What would they like? Would they like such and such? Always **ask** the patient's opinion and approval. Also, most providers left Mom "uncovered" after checking her. She was left undignified and cold. She said that she felt like she had been thrown around like a piece of meat. One doctor sat and looked her in the eyes, made her smile and spoke to her as a human being. It meant the world to her. The smallest things are important to maintaining self-respect and dignity.
- Ensure the patient's right to evaluate every option, with the known benefits and risks. **All treatment options should be presented**, not just the ones that a provider

thinks are useful.

- Encourage providers to evaluate your situation based on your unique circumstances, to creatively think beyond protocols.
- Be open to complementary treatment modalities such as massage, acupuncture, Feldenkrais, and many others.
- Continue to evaluate new treatment options. Even if the current treatment plan is working, ask your medical provider if there is any new treatment available and present any new treatment you hear about to them.

Other:
- Ensure that all insurance claims and provider payments are tracked. Insurance is constantly changing and bills are often wrong.

After everything that I experienced, I personally will not leave anyone that I love and care about in the hospital or a care facility alone if their condition is critical or if they are unable to advocate for themself. When my mom was in critical condition or recently out of surgery, my sisters and I would take shifts and stay with her around the clock to advocate for her care and safety. Once she was stable and able to advocate for herself, we would have her caregivers stay with her, allowing us to go home and rest knowing that we would be called if needed. Because my dad was unable to advocate for himself, due to having Alzheimer's, when he was hospitalized or in a care facility, a family member or trusted caregiver would stay with him at all times.

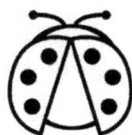

Let me fall if I must.
The one I will become will catch me.
Baal Shem Tov

Chapter 3

MANAGING CARE ...
preparation and thriving in the blur

You have responded to the request to manage the care of another. You may recall from Chapter 1 that author and disability rights advocate Richard Pimentel defines responsibility as responding to your ability. You may have decided to oversee the care and to delegate many of the necessary daily management tasks. But for purposes of this book, I will proceed as though you responded with willingness to at minimum actively manage the care of another person.

As with all new responsibilities, especially one which may involve times of crisis, it can become a blur. The road of managing care can be long and sometimes a bit unforgiving, causing us to go into mental overload.

Possibly the biggest challenge you will face in managing the care of another is gathering and organizing information so that it is easily accessible, always current and effectively disseminated. While your situation will be unique, I will share what was useful in helping my family stay on top of care management.

Know Your Rights and Those of the Patient
If you have been asked to manage care for another, it is important to know what your responsibilities and rights are. Will you actively be the medical power of attorney? If not, will that power be given to you at some future time? If the

person requiring your assistance is still in control of their own decisions, will they work with you so that you can effectively oversee their care? What are they asking you to do? Whatever your situation, you need to be clear about what the patient wants you to do and what authority you have to do it. (See *Peaceful Endings*, Chapter 2, Power of Attorney and *Peaceful Endings*, Afterword, *What You Need to Do to Create a Will*.)

It is also important to know the rights of the person for whom you are managing care. For example, they have the right to multiple medical opinions, informed consent, to refuse treatment and to refuse to be taken to an ED. There are many federal and state laws that protect those rights and many others. A professional patient advocate can be of assistance with this information.

The Almighty Emergency Information Book
If an Emergency Information Book does not already exist, create it NOW!

- Get a three-ring notebook and some paper. *We chose red so that it was easy to find in an emergency.*
- Gather the information below and put it in the notebook.
- Label the notebook "Emergency Information Book".
- Keep the book in a specific place in the home or facility and be sure that everyone involved with care knows what and where it is.
- Be clear that **the book is to go to with the patient every time they go to the ED or hospital**.

The contents of the Emergency Information Book are as follows:

🐞🐞🐞 Keep this book up-to-date at all times!

- Emergency contacts: name, relationship and phone number for each
- Medical power of attorney: name and phone number, including documentation that supports the designation for each (a copy)
- Medical history – summary, listing past medical issues and current health details, especially any recent hospitalizations or episodes
- Family medical history
- Allergies
- Current prescription medicines, and any over-the-counter products and supplements: name, dosage and schedule of administration
- Physicians: primary care and all specialists listing name, and phone number
- Advance directives (a copy)
- Do Not Resuscitate order, if applicable
- Medical insurance cards – private, Medicare and secondary, or Medicaid (a copy)
- Driver's license or government issued id (a copy)

🐞🐞 I would recommend that you have a couple of copies of any documents that you might hand over to the hospital admissions staff, such as an id and medical insurance cards. While the intention is for them to copy and return your document, that sometimes does not happen and you end up with a document missing from your book.

🐞🐞 Another practice is to *always verify and update* the contents of your Emergency Information Book upon returning home from the episode.

The Best 99-Cent Investment

The spiral notebook is the best 99-cent investment a care management team can make. Buy a half dozen, you will probably need them all and may need more.

Each time Mom and Dad started a new medical episode, requiring treatment for either a new condition or one unrelated to a previous episode, we started to use a *new spiral notebook*. We wrote the date and episode type (location such as hospital or diagnosis) on the front. From that point on, we documented everything that happened in regard to that episode.

It was a running log of all conversations and interactions with medical providers, all appointments, and of course all visits to the ED and admissions to the hospital.

Whichever family member or caregiver was responsible for overseeing an event (an appointment, conversation, time in the hospital), would start a new page in the notebook and list the day, time, and who was taking the notes. That person then documented *everything*: who entered the room; who said what and to whom; anything done to the patient, including basic care such as a bed bath; any procedure performed; the administration of medications, including IVs; and any therapy, etc. We created a running log of all activity. We even logged what time a meal was ordered, if it arrived, and how much was eaten. It may seem like overkill, but when you are in a medical crisis, you may not remember whether you ordered the meal or if it arrived. Additionally, we had a system of highlighting particularly important information, especially changes to medications, so that those reading the notes in the future would be sure to notice the change.

As I said in the beginning, at some point things will become a blur. Information that seems understood and clear in the moment is often unretrievable after the fact. The spiral notebooks were always available to family and caregivers so that they could read the most current medical treatment and care information. The notebooks were essential in reducing the number of times information had to be repeated to family members and caregivers. The logs also reduced the number of calls to medical providers to verify information and prevented multiple family members from asking providers the same question.

When we utilized the spiral notebooks in a hospital or facility, we were sometimes initially met by providers with a somewhat negative curiosity. Some of the medical providers were fearful that we were documenting things which might cause them trouble. We quickly learned to assure them that we were documenting things in order to retain quickly changing information; to keep our large family and caregiver team up-to-date; and to prevent our group from arriving and asking questions that had already been answered.

We also shared that we used the notebooks to create a collective list of all of our questions. That way, whoever was present when the medical providers arrived had a collective list of everyone's questions. The answers were then written by the questions so that our group could find them.

🐞🐞 Sometimes we blocked out a section on a page, in the midst of our notes, for questions and their answers and dog-eared the page for easy access. Often we used a colored highlighter to box the section so that it was visibly different. Other times we saved the pages at the back of the spiral notebook for questions and their answers. Always the Q&A sections were dated and signed by the person who asked the questions and wrote the answers.

After a while, the doctors and RNs began to occasionally rely on us for the most current information. If a doctor wanted to know when the last IV was changed or what the last test result was, and an RN was unavailable, they knew that we could provide the information immediately.

An unexpected value of the notebooks came when a new episode started and we could not remember which medication had previously caused an adverse reaction. If we were in the same hospital as the previous episode, they might have a record of it. (We learned that they also might not have a record of it.) If not, we were on our own to remember... and the spiral notebooks became invaluable! We also found that many times the history we documented allowed us to identify the cause of seemingly "random" or unexplainable symptoms. By looking back at our extremely detailed notes, we were able to identify a pattern or the relationship of an event to a symptom which was not identifiable by medical providers.

A Library of Notebooks

Initially the Emergency Information Book and the spiral notebooks were all that we needed. But as medical needs escalated, I quickly found the need to develop a library of three ring notebooks, each labeled for a specific type of information associated with my parents' care. There was a notebook for:

- Medical papers such as test results and instructions for procedures (Although many are now online, we still kept hard copy, which was the method my parents preferred.)
- Insurance policies – secondary and long-term care
- Medical insurance claims, to both Medicare and secondary insurance
- Long-term care insurance terms and claims
- Legal documents such as power of attorney designation, advance directive, last will and testament, trust documents and DNR if applicable
- Household bills and payments
- Information on caregiver services including information about agencies, registries and independent caregiver sources (See Chapter 8.)
- Independent caregiver applications and documentation
- Information on facilities such as skilled rehabilitation: including administration personnel list, policies, patient commitments, your pre-meeting notes, their meeting notes (which you will have signed), any daily log sheets and a copy of their medication administration list
- Information on palliative and hospice care services (See *Peaceful Endings*.)

And as my parents' care needs increased, and we chose to bring caregivers into their home, the need for additional notebooks arose:
- A Caregiver Book
- Daily Log Sheets
- Shift-Turnover Sheets
- Care Team Newsletters
- Caregiver paycards

(See Chapter 9.)

The Web of Communication

In *Peaceful Endings*, Chapter 1, Sharing Information, I discuss the challenges of sharing information, in regard to a diagnosis and the overall status of the patient, with friends and family. In this situation there is always a choice of if and how much information is shared, allowing for control of whether the sharing is energizing or depleting. In the coordination of care management, however, detailed information must be shared efficiently and effectively. That communication can be very time consuming and depleting.

In my situation, my sisters and I utilized all methods of communication. A conference call was used when a situation was urgent and/or if the originator was driving. Text threads were for updates, and emails were used for lengthy communication. Sometimes a text was used to let the group know that an email had been sent and needed attention. Emails received regarding care could be stored in a separate email folder for easy access. And an important email could also be printed and put in a notebook for quick reference in the future.

Sometimes we took photos of pages in the spiral notebooks containing new information and texted them to each other, saving us the time required to retype the information or to repeat it verbally.

Time Flies

When I was in grade school, the days seemed to last forever. I actually remember wondering how I was ever going to get to be a teenager. Now I am continually amazed at how quickly time passes. This is particularly true when you enter the bubble of managing care. When my care managing responsibilities ended nearly 2 ½ years after they started, I could hardly believe that much time had passed. It had gone in a heartbeat. During that time, I would try to remember in what year some event took place, and I simply couldn't. It was all a blur with all the years running into each other.

There are several ways to help keep the events of each year separate in your mind, including making a list of occurrences with dates. Because I am very visual, I found the circle method helpful. Each circle represents a year, with the year the experience started in the middle.

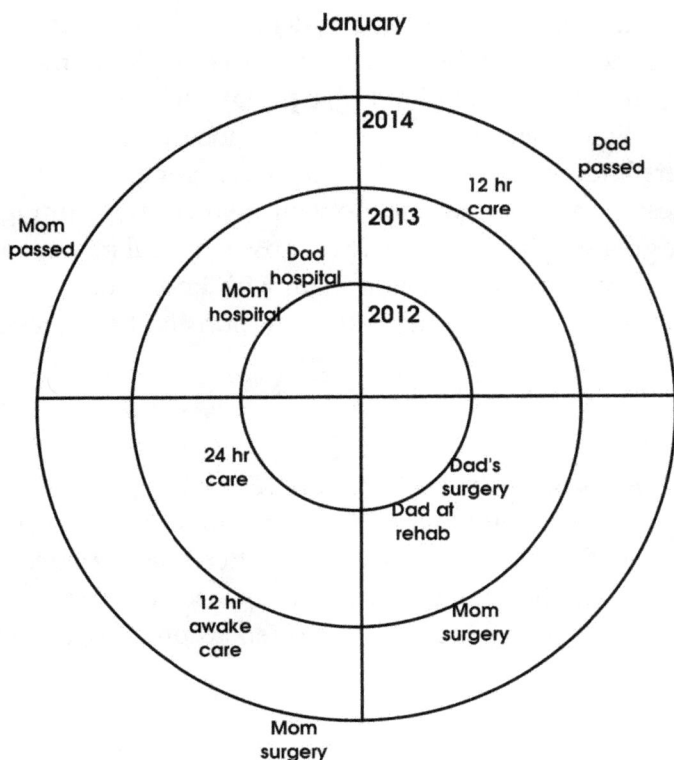

The Second Wave

There will come a time when you have gathered and organized the information necessary for the immediate care needs, and you can take a breath. You may be lucky enough to coast for a while in a stable care situation, or you may only have a moment to regroup before another part of the journey is presented. In either case, you are probably at the beginning of a much longer journey for which you need to prepare.

Peaceful Endings not only provides additional information needed for crisis management but also explains the fundamentals of estate planning and estate settlement. We all face death. Everyone must understand the steps that will ensure our end-of-life needs or our loved one's are met and decisions honored. Find out if any estate planning has been done. Find out where essential documents are and understand them. And after you have gone through the process for your loved one, do your own estate planning. It is the greatest gift you can give to those who will manage and provide care for you, leaving them with knowledge of what you want and relieving them of the responsibility of guessing your desires.

An Experiment in In-DEPENDENCE

When managing another's care, it is important that you do your best to understand what the other is experiencing. I don't mean the actual illness or disease, but rather the limitations and dependence that often accompany the need for care.

After I had finished providing care for my parents, someone told me about a program in which they were required to do an experiment in how it felt to give up a piece of their independence, to be dependent on another person. Their experience required them to live blindfolded for a period of time. I thought about it and played with it, but ultimately I was unnerved by the inconvenience of dependency.

A year ago I was struggling with unexplained bouts of vertigo. The most recent, and hopefully last, bout resulted in my inability to stand. For the better part of a week I was unable to walk unattended or freely. It was an interesting lesson in how it feels to be reliant on another for basic needs. Even though I knew that eventually I would be well and independent, it was an invaluable experience in the need for understanding and compassion when dependent.

> I've learned that
> people will forget what you said,
> people will forget what you did,
> but people will never forget
> how you made them feel.
> Maya Angelou

I learned that beyond the frustration of not being able to do what I had previously taken for granted, there was a sensitivity in my willingness to accept unsolicited help. The use of "May I?" by any person offering assistance, as opposed to assuming my acceptance, was powerful and an invaluable lesson.

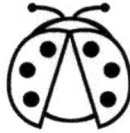

People who need help
sometimes look a lot like
people who don't need help.
Glennon Melton

Chapter 4

IDENTIFYING CARE NEEDS ...
ADLs, IADLS and the "three big killers"

The need to manage a person's care likely will develop in one of several ways. My parents' need for and acceptance of care was more evolutionary than revolutionary. In the beginning it involved doing little chores such as changing all the burned out lightbulbs, fixing things and running errands during each visit from out of state. For many years my sister who lived near my parents provided increasing oversight and assistance when necessary. Over time my visits became more frequent and my sisters and I gradually provided more assistance, which was offered delicately and given only when accepted. Once my dad experienced a medical crisis, requiring months of 24-hour oversight, the stage was set for full-time care without resistance. From that point, the need for a care team developed quickly.

For other people, the care need arises suddenly, leaving no time for a family member to prepare or ease into the new role of care manager or caregiver. Loved ones may realize the need for care before the person living with the medical issues faces their need. Sometimes the person living with the medical issues acknowledges the need for care. That acknowledgement greatly simplifies the process of providing care. In situations when a loved one does not acknowledge their need for care, it can be more difficult to step into the role of care manager or provider. At some point in every situation, there will be a need to identify the care needs of another and to develop a care plan to address those needs.

In all situations, it is helpful to know the patient's philosophy of and goal for medical treatment and care. For example, my parents' goal was to preserve quality of life instead of striving purely for longevity. We also knew our parents' wishes for treatment at each stage of the care process. This allowed our parents to make decisions by evaluating each option based on their goal. It also guided us in providing their care.

Determining Care Needs

The language of "activities of daily living" helps determine care requirements and the level of coverage that will address them. An assessment of those requirements facilitates talking about them. There are two types of activities of daily living. First, there are the activities required for basic health and survival. Then there are activities that contribute to quality of life and independence.

Activities of Daily Living

ADLs are basic self-care tasks that are learned as a child and are required for basic health and survival. An assessment of a person's ability to do the following tasks without assistance can determine the level of care they require. Long-term care insurance policies mandate that a patient require assistance with two or more ADLs before a claim for benefits can be made. They consist of:

1. Bathing/showering
2. Personal hygiene and grooming
   Brushing/combing hair, oral care
3. Dressing
4. Toilet hygiene
   Getting on/off, cleaning oneself, including continence

5. Functional mobility or transferring
   Walking, getting into and out of a bed and chair
6. Self-feeding

Instrumental Activities of Daily Living
IADLs are tasks that contribute to a person's quality of life and their ability to live independently. An assessment of a person's ability to do the following tasks without assistance can determine whether the person can safely live independently or if they need assistance with specific activities occasionally. Depending on the tasks that require assistance, more constant oversight may be necessary. They are:

1. Managing finances
   Bill payment, managing banking accounts, managing financial planning
2. Handling transportation
   Driving or navigating public transportation or getting rides
3. Shopping
   Food and errands
4. Preparing meals
5. Using communication devices
6. Managing medications
   Administering, reordering
7. Housework and basic home maintenance
8. Pet care, if applicable

I would add to these standard IADLs, an evaluation of
9. Health care management
   Medical appointments, insurance claim management
10. Legal management
    Execution and maintenance of legal documents

The "Three Big Killers"

In *A Most Meaningful Life*, Chapter 10, *The Real Killers* I reference the book *Learning from Hannah, Secrets for a Life Worth Living* by William H Thomas. This book identifies the "three big killers" of the aging as:

helplessness, loneliness and hopelessness.

In addition to the ADLs and IADLs, it is important to evaluate a person's susceptibility to the three big killers, as they may be as big a threat to the person's quality of life, health, safety and comfort as any serious medical condition or limitation.

Helplessness is often experienced as a person begins to require –but often does not want - assistance, and perceives that they are losing their independence. Creating an environment that allows them to do as much as possible for themselves maintains their feeling of self-worth, and deters a feeling of helplessness.

Another significant issue is the *loneliness* that stems from social isolation as a person loses mobility and independence. Family members often are geographically dispersed and unable to assist with care. In a Forbes.com article titled *Loneliness Might Be a Bigger Health Risk Than Smoking or Obesity*, writer Brad Porter examines the impact of loneliness on health. The article, which was published Jan. 18, 2017, cites a Brigham Young University study that found that isolation increases the risk of death by 30%, with some saying as much as 60%. "To put it another way, loneliness might be a more significant health factor than obesity, smoking, exercise or nutrition." Besides causing psychological symptoms (such as depression) and having practical or circumstantial effects (such as not getting the help necessary to keep someone safe), there is evidence that loneliness has a negative physiological impact on the body (such as depressing the immune system) in a manner similar to stress. Simply, loneliness can result in death.

It is important to ensure that the person whose mobility and independence are decreasing will be where people can engage with them and they will be encouraged to engage with others, staving off loneliness.

The third danger, *hopelessness,* can be the result of helplessness and loneliness. By preventing feelings of helplessness and loneliness; ensuring quality of life; and providing things to look forward to, such as visits and outings, hopelessness should be avoided.

The "three big killers" lead to depression, apathy, loss of self-worth and, therefore, loss of a reason to live. Avoiding the three big killers is as important to the care and well-being of an individual as administering medication and keeping them safe and comfortable.

Assistance with Needs Assessment
If you need assistance in evaluating the person's needs, a medical professional, physical or occupational therapist, or social worker can help.

In addition, every county in the United States is required by federal law to provide information about and assist with access to senior services. These vary and may include case management, which may encompass a comprehensive needs assessment and care-plan development. They also offer other services that may be needed after an initial needs assessment and care plan have been developed. These may include assistance with locating appropriate care, the loaning of assistive devices, transportation options and more. Some counties provide services for multiple counties and share resources. Google: "find local Area Agency on Aging" followed by the zipcode or county and state or visit http://www.n4a.org. Otherwise, call your county and ask to be directed to the senior services department.

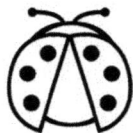

Home is not a place ... it is a feeling.
Unknown

Chapter 5

HOUSING OPTIONS ...
finding the best fit

The first step in creating a care plan is to determine the best housing option for the person. The best option may be their current housing, or they may need to move. That decision should be based on the care-needs assessment, which encompasses ADLs and IADLs; availability of resources for care needs; the person's ability to be kept safe but comfortable; and the opportunity for a good quality of life.

Each Housing Option Has a Purpose
Understanding the various housing alternatives is the first step in determining the best option.

Staying at home is just that: the person lives in their home, independently and with minimal care needs. It may be in a single-family home, condo or apartment. Home modifications and some assistive devices, such as a walker, can make a home safer and extend the time before additional assistance is needed.

A ***senior-living community*** (usually 55 or 62 years of age and older) or living independently in a ***continuing-care retirement community (CCRC)*** offer the opportunity to interact and socialize with the availability of some services, such as meal preparation, transportation and event planning.

Once a person living independently needs assistance or care, they can consider hiring **nonmedical home-care services** to assist with ADLs and IADLs. These services can be obtained by contracting with a home-care agency or registry or by employing independent caregivers. (See Chapter 8.) At this point, they also may consider moving in with a family member or into one of the living situations described below.

Assisted living emphasizes quality of life and independence while offering some care and assistance with ADLs. On the care spectrum, this level of care is between independent living and skilled nursing, and may be available in a CCRC, an assisted-living community or an assisted-living residential home.

Memory care offers those with dementia and other memory deficits specialized care and a safe environment. Those working in memory care have specialized training. While there are facilities and communities dedicated to memory care, some CCRCs, assisted-living communities and assisted-living residential homes offer sections of their facilities that provide memory-care services.

Skilled nursing is sometimes associated with housing, as it is often an offering at a CCRC or senior-living community. However, it is a *type of service* which may be required after a medical crisis or injury, or as medical care needs increase. The *goal* of skilled nursing is to provide temporary care allowing the patient *to return to original housing or an option requiring less care.* Occasionally an SNF becomes a long-term residence, a form of housing, and is sometimes referred to as a nursing home.

CCRCs and senior-living communities offer varying options for housing and care including independent living, assisted living, memory care and skilled nursing.

With the growth of the senior population in the United States, there is a growing concern over finding suitable, affordable housing for this demographic. The need for finding new housing options is paramount. Websites, such as APlaceForMom.com, assist in the search for senior-care services. There are an increasing number of creative housing options available as well. *"Granny pods,"* small individual housing units, are now available for purchase and placement in a back yard. There are efforts to create *"pocket neighborhoods"* of small homes for seniors who can share skills and assist each other. *"Co-housing"* is an intentional community of private homes clustered around shared space. *Shared living* includes *home sharing* with a roommate and *group homes,* a new twist on boardinghouses, and is a term that is becoming popular to describe multiple adult friends sharing one home. Some group homes offer independent living and others offer assisted-living care assistance.

AARP's *Livable Communities* (www.aarp.org/livable-communities/about) supports the efforts of communities in providing livable places for people of all ages and life stages. It provides helpful information regarding what to look for in a community, as well as a Livability Index that rates a community as to how livable it is in regard to aging. Its objective is to assist seniors in identifying communities in which they can "age in place." For example, if a senior cannot drive, they need a community that offers transportation options.

The *Village to Village Network* (www.vtvnetwork.clubexpress.com) helps communities establish and manage their own ***aging in place initiatives*** called Villages. A Village is a membership-driven, nonprofit organization that coordinates access to affordable services, including some volunteer services, and access to providers who are vetted and offer services at a discount. The objective is to allow members to age safely and successfully in their own homes.

As the senior population continues to grow, there is no doubt there will be many other initiatives to assist in aging at home.

🐞🐞 All of the terms bolded in this section can be used in a Google search to find more information.

Considerations When Moving Seniors

I moved to Denver from the home which I had custom built and in which I had raised my daughter, met and married my husband, spent time with his two children, loved two dogs and built a life. As I was packing and leaving, I was sad. My daughter, then 25 said to me, "Don't be sad, the memories are not in the house, they are in your heart." True and sage advice to remember, as one day we may all face the need to move into different housing or a care facility to meet our needs.

My parents wanted to live independently in their own home until the end of their lives. Over time, my family assisted my parents in making small modifications to the home to accommodate that goal. Many years after my dad was diagnosed with Alzheimer's, it became unsafe for him to continue living in a two-story home. My mom immediately found an alternative: a single-level condo into which she could move all of their belongings in order to recreate the home that they loved. I will forever feel that their willingness to move into a safer home in which my sisters and I could help them live for the remainder of their lives was one of the greatest gifts that they gave me. I know that my mom made the decision to move partly for their safety, but also because she understood that it would make the lives of me and my sisters easier as we accepted more responsibility for their care. For that too, I will always be grateful.

It is understandable that some people are very attached to their single-family homes and the independence they feel there. While no one should be forced to move, they can be delicately encouraged to do so if their health and safety are at stake. Keep in mind that there often is a window of opportunity to make a move. As care needs increase and mobility decreases, it becomes harder to make a transition and assimilate into the new environment. The sooner a move to a long-term housing situation can be made, the easier it is on everyone. It will not only help them to live more comfortably, but help family and other caregivers provide the best possible care for them. If a senior refuses to move and the situation is unsafe, contact your county for resources that may be helpful.

Relocation Stress Syndrome and Transfer Trauma
It has long been said that the relocation of an elderly person can have adverse effects. The term *relocation stress* may be defined as a state in which an individual experiences negative physical effects and/or mental disturbances as a result of transferring from one environment to another. *Transfer anxiety,* causing depression and potentially elevated morbidity rates, is caused by the separation from a known and secure environment to an unknown environment or from the perception of the move as negative. While studies

vary, many indicate a relationship between transferring patients and increases in post-transfer morbidity and mortality risks.

That is not to say that older adults should not be relocated. However, the decision to move them should be based on necessity, and the move must be handled with care. As with many aspects of care, finesse can be used to frame the move in a positive light. Every effort should be made to see that the actual moving process is as stress free as possible for the person, physically and psychologically. Care should be taken to allay any fears that the person may have about moving. One of those fears may be related to the disposition of their personal property.

Personal Property
Their possessions are theirs, not yours. Every generation is different in how they perceive personal belongings. My parents' generation, having lived through the Great Depression and World War II, had to struggle and sacrifice for everything that they owned. They valued possessions, took great care of them and wanted to pass their treasured items to the next generation. Many of today's millennials are minimalists and are not interested in inheriting items from previous generations.

None of that gives anyone the right to dispose of the property of another person without their permission. It is disrespectful and can be distressing. I have witnessed all too many times a child who takes over the care of their parent and then immediately begins to dispose of their possessions. In many cases, those possessions anchor their owner to reality.

If the person is moving to smaller quarters, work with them to make decisions about their property. If that is not immediately possible, consider temporarily placing the excess items into a storage unit until after the person has adjusted to the relocation.

Matching Housing to Needs

My parents always knew that they wanted to remain at home for their entire lives. They had no desire to move to a senior-living community as they had each other and their family for socialization and care. Sadly, my dad previously had ushered all of his friends through their final days, but my mom continued to see her girlfriends, one from kindergarten (via facetime), a few from college and her best friend with whom she shared 84 years of friendship. Both had visits from their three daughters, three sons-in-law, 7 grandchildren, 3 great grandchildren and an occasional dog. In addition, at one time we had a crew of 7 additional caregivers in and out of the house in any given week.

Following are three other situations that demonstrate the difficulty of the housing decision:

My childhood friend provided care for her mother. She lived in a large house in which the two bedrooms at the far end of the upstairs could be converted to a bedroom and a living room/kitchen. Her mother loved to cook and therefore, my friend had a "fancy" kitchen installed for her mother. My friend and her husband lived in the home with their three children. They thought it was the best housing choice for her mother. While it was a more convenient way to look after her mother, my friend said, in retrospect, she felt that her mother had been lonely. It was possible that socialization

71

might have been more important than convenience and a nice kitchen, and that another choice might have provided more socialization for her mother. Hindsight can seem perfect, but remember that we can only make the best decision based on the information we have at the time.

Another friend is faced with housing needs for both of her parents who have long been divorced. Her father is a man with increasing care needs, few financial resources and some behaviors that will make it challenging to find housing. In contrast, her mother has financial resources, requires care, lives with hoarding disorder and is unwilling to move from her home.

My mom's sister moved across the country to be near a son who was to oversee her increasing care needs. She moved into independent living and within two years was in need of assisted living. After several falls and serious injuries, and inadequate care oversight, she was moved back to the area where she had resided for many years. One of her daughters now can oversee the care provided by an assisted-living facility and offer more family support and socialization.

The point is that there are as many unique situations as there are people. Some people can and want to be at home. Others want the socialization and services offered by a community environment. There is no one right option, but instead possibly only the best option for the individual. And that option may require re-evaluation and change over time.

Chapter 4 provides information on how to get assistance with the needs assessment. The Seniors Blue Book, resources for aging well, provides many helpful resources (www.SeniorsBlueBook.com).

When considering housing options, assess each option and your ability to keep the home safe (see below.)

1. Assess the current environment.
   Assess the person's openness to accepting help in this environment in the future, if necessary.

2. Evaluate housing alternatives.
   Services such as Caring.com, APlaceforMom.com and the Seniors Blue Book are just some of the places in which you can find direction on housing options in your area. Google some of the terms identified in *Each Housing Option Has a Purpose* above.

   🐞🐞🐞 Be clear on what the option does and does not provide and at what cost.

   🐞🐞 When evaluating other options, especially when falling is a concern, know that there may be an assumption that moving a person to assisted living will *eliminate* the falls. It is not inherently true. Any housing alternative that promises to eliminate falls, without assigning someone to monitor a person 24x7, is not being honest. A person who falls while in assisted living may be found sooner than someone living independently, which may result in them receiving potentially life-saving treatment sooner. That said, alternative-housing options may be better equipped to monitor the safety of the environment and ensure things like proper medication administration, which help to *prevent* falls.

3. Consider the impact on everyone involved.

   What really is the best environment for the person, one with options for socialization with peers or one that offers geographic proximity to family? If family members are going to be caregiving, accessibility is a greater consideration.

4. Consider finances.

   It is critical to evaluate the financial situation. Key factors in assessing the financial situation are the age and health status of the person, the person's assets and any other sources of support. Determine whether there are unclaimed benefits, such as those for veterans, which can now be utilized. Are there long-term care benefits that can be initiated at some point? Depending on your specific situation, it may be helpful to contact a financial planner for the assessment. In doing this assessment, it is important to fully understand all of the expenses involved with each option being considered.

   👀👀👀 While various housing options offer many services, there is a cost for each of them. Some options offer all services in a package price, others are a la carte and are very expensive. Be sure you know the real costs, as well as how the costs for providing those services in a private setting would compare.

Assessing the Current Environment

According to a survey by Home Instead Senior Care, "85% of seniors have done nothing to prepare their home for aging." Their research also says that 33% of trips to the ER are caused by accidents at home, 48% of which could have been prevented. Although emergency department doctors

74

say that it's very important that families invest in basic home safety modifications, very few do so.

Once identified, there are many modifications that can be made for little or no cost. A small investment in modifications may prevent an injury and resultant medical bills or even delay a costly future move.

Keep in mind your person's specific circumstances. Walk through the environment envisioning what life would be like if you lived there with any ailments they may have, such as arthritis or diminished eyesight, hearing or mobility.

Following are things to consider when assessing the current housing environment. *It is not all inclusive but covers many safety concerns. Hopefully this list will get you thinking and you will identify more areas to evaluate.* Some of these may not be immediately relevant but over time should be examined.

In general:
- Clutter
  Is there clutter? If there is, can it be organized? Can additional storage, such as shelves, be installed? Can it be cleaned out? (See the caution about Personal Property above.)

- Furniture
  o Is there too much furniture? Is it posing a safety hazard, specifically the risk of falling? Keep in mind that some furniture is used for stabilization as the person walks through a room. Watch the person maneuver through their space to determine if this is the case.

o   Is the furniture stable? If not, can it be repaired?
o   Are the chairs the right height for the person? Are the person's knees above their hips when sitting? If so, the chair is too low and a pillow can be added to raise the seat height. Do the person's feet touch the ground? If not, the chair is too high for the person and should possibly be replaced. Are the chair legs and arms sturdy or do they need repair?
o   Is the bed too low (knees are above hips when sitting on the edge of the bed)? If so, bed raisers can be put under the feet of the bed. Is the bed too high (feet don't touch the floor when legs are over the side of the bed)? If so, can the bed frame be removed and/or can a lower-profile mattress be used?

- Flooring
  o   Is the wall-to-wall carpeting easy to walk on? Are there rumples that could be professionally stretched out? Are there tears that need to be repaired? Can it, should it, be removed?
  o   Are there throw carpets? If so, remove them.
  o   Where there is no carpeting, is the flooring slippery? Can a nonstick cleaning product be applied? Can the person wear nonskid shoes and socks when shoeless?

- Doorways
  o   Do the doorway openings restrict the ability of a walker to pass through? If so, consider having swing-clear hinges installed that will add up to 2 additional inches of pass through clearance to the door opening.
  o   Are there door thresholds? Are they a tripping hazard? Can they be removed?

- Lighting

  Is the light sufficient for safety, including in closets and pantries? Can the wattage of bulbs be increased to allowable limits? Can lamps be added or overhead lighting be installed? Can under-counter lighting, utilizing battery-operated pucks, be added? Would the use of a Clapper or other device to assist with turning lights on and off, be helpful? Would light timers be helpful, especially when entering the home at night? Could rope lighting be run between a bedroom to a bathroom to show the way at night? Can nightlights be placed in sockets in all hallways and throughout the living space? Would motion activated lights be helpful, especially in the bedroom and bathroom?

- Cabinet accessibility

  Are contents of cabinets accessible? Are they too high or too low? Would in-cabinet organizers be helpful? The use of a Lazy Susan inside a cabinet, on a countertop, and/or in the fridge can be helpful.

- Electrical cords

  Are electrical cords organized and safely out of any path? Can a power strip be used or items moved to minimize electrical cords being exposed?

- Alarms
  - Is there a smoke detector/alarm on every floor and outside every bedroom? Are the batteries current? Batteries need to be changed annually – pick a birthday and do it.
  - Is there a carbon monoxide detector? Does it have an audible alarm?

- Faucets
    - Are the faucets single-lever style? If not, replace them as they are easier than twist knobs and safer in mixing the cold and hot water.
    - Check the hot water temperature. Consider setting it to 120 degrees. If you have separate hot and cold water faucets, consider marking them with red and blue to identify the hot and cold. Some older homes have the knobs reversed, which poses a safety risk.

- Stairs
  Is there a railing the length of the wall? Are there one or two railings? Can an additional railing be installed if necessary? Is the bottom stair identified in some way? Is there a nonslip surface: adhesive stair tread or carpet? Are the stairs clear of clutter?

  👓👓 There are in-home alternatives for stairs. An AssiStep *stair walker* (www.Assistep.com) provides support in front of a person when walking up or down stairs. A *stairlift* is a mechanical device for lifting people up and down stairs. They are available for straight and curved staircases; are made for both inside and outdoor use; and offer the option for lifting people in wheelchairs. A *home elevator* eliminates the need to use stairs. It may be a better option for someone in a wheelchair. While these options may not be inexpensive, in the long run it may be cost-effective if it can keep a person in their home. Google: your city or state followed by "stair walker," "stairlift" or "home elevator."

- Doorbell
  Does the doorbell ring loudly enough to be heard? If not, consider installing a doorbell that triggers a flashing light to indicate that it has been rung.

- Outdoors
  - Garage: Is the overhead garage door always kept down? Is the overhead door operated with an electric door opener? If there is a separate door to the garage, is it locked?
  - Are all windows closed when the home is left?
  - Is yard work (lawn cut, bushes trimmed, snow removed, pet poop removed) maintained? If not, how will this happen?
  - Is there outdoor lighting? If so, are the bulbs working? Consider adding motion-activated lighting.

- Bathrooms
  - Grab bars
    Are there grab bars near the tub, shower, and toilet? If not, have them installed. Towel bars and curtain rods are not grab bars and should not be used as such.
  - Tub/shower
    - Is the tub too low or too high? Consider using a tub transfer bench. There are devices available that will lower and raise a body in and out of the tub. There are also walk in tubs.
    - Is the tub/shower slippery? There are nonslip, stick-on decals, but I have found *Tub Grip Clear anti-slip bathroom coating by Grip-It* to be the most reliable product. I do not recommend using a suction on bath mat because they often don't stick.

- Is there a bench in the tub/shower?
  - Is the showerhead wall-mounted? Consider replacing it with a hand-held unit, mounting the head at an easily reachable height and allowing it to be used as a showerhead or hand-held sprayer.
  - Toilets
    Is the toilet the correct height? If it is too low (knees are above hips when seated), a toilet riser can be added. If the toilet is too high, consider replacing it. Comfort height toilets, 17", are now available.

- Other safety considerations
  - Is there at least one fire extinguisher? One should be easily accessible from the kitchen.
  - Is there a reaching device to assist with retrieving items that have fallen?
  - Is a walker used? Are there rubber tips on the walker? If the walker has wheels, are there tennis ball glides on the other ends?
  - Is there a table or counter by the main entrance, to set things on while entering the home? This allows the person to immediately lock the door behind them before proceeding into the home with their items.
  - Are there containers into which products such as laundry detergent can be divided for easier lifting?
  - Can medications be managed safely and accurately? Where are they stored? Are they accessible? Who monitors them? Having prescriptions filled and packaged by Pillpack.com or using an organizer for pills may be helpful.
  - Is there easy access to a phone, particularly during the night? Is there a cordless or wireless option? Is emergency information easily available? Would a phone specifically designed to work well with

hearing aids be helpful? Would an emergency alert device be useful? Would a phone with a larger visual display and keypad or a louder volume be helpful?

- <u>Important items</u>
  - o Are important (purse/wallet, checkbook) items stored in a place where they can always be found?
  - o Is emergency contact information visible on the refrigerator?
  - o Has an Emergency Information Book been created? (See Chapter 3.) Is it where the purse/wallet is stored?

Evaluating Housing Alternatives

After assessing the current housing environment and determining whether modifications are possible when necessary, it is time to evaluate housing alternatives. Even if the current housing option continues to be feasible, it may not be the best option available or may not be a long-term option. It is wise to continue the evaluation process by, at minimum, gathering basic information such as locations and costs of alternatives. When possible, conduct an assessment similar to that which you did for the current environment. It will aid in validating a choice to remain in the current housing situation as well as in planning for future needs.

👓👓 Www.APlaceForMom.com and www.Caring.com are two websites that provide assistance with identifying housing and care options. You can also Google: your city or state followed by any of the housing types, such as "assisted living."

The use of a grid or spreadsheet to track information may be helpful. Below is an example of a grid on which not only services and costs can be tracked but also proximity to family. Specific features such as meal preparation, transportation and community events can be noted.

	Housing Comparison Grid								
	Location	Type of Housing (H, Ind, AS)	Proximity to Manager	Proximity to Advocate	Cost of Independent Housing	Cost of Assisted Living Housing	Cost of Assistance with ADLs	Cost of Assistance With IADLs	Cost of Additional Services
1									
	Notes:								
2									
	Notes:								
3									
	Notes:								
4									
	Notes:								

You will also want to compare the cost of all housing options and the amount of care they provide. The following chart shows some relative costs, for example purposes only. In my family's case, it was not only what my parents wanted but also less expensive to provide care for them in their home. Their home expenses were minimal.

Housing/Care Comparison
relative cost comparison for example purposes only

Home *	CCRC **	Assisted Living	Private Room Nursing Home	Semi-private Nursing Home
$164.00	$166.67	$200.00	$712.25	$638.58
$4,920.00	$5,000.00	$6,000.00	$8,547.00	$7,663.00
$59,040.00	$60,000.00	$72,000.00	$102,564.00	$91,956.00

*** Memory Care is an additional cost.

* Home
This represents the cost of in-home care.
Other home costs must be added.

** CCRCs, *independent living with no care services*
$5,000 is a average as the cost of CCRC living is extremely variable.
National averages for CCRCs range from $2800 - $9000.
Some offer a la carte services and are all-inclusive.
Some CCRC's offer rentals and others require entry fees with a significant investment.

Making a Housing Decision

The decision-making process is never easy, as it may involve change. There are countless considerations in selecting housing. The best that you can do for another is to research the alternatives, identify the pros and cons of each, and then present the options.

All the discussions about housing and care require compassion and finesse. No one, of any age, likes to feel that they are being told what to do or that they have lost control of their independence or decisions. The more the person whose housing needs are being evaluated can be involved in the process, the smoother the process should go. Once you have your grid of information it is time to discuss the information. Empower the person by being clear that you have facilitated the gathering of information so that the person can make an informed decision. The decision belongs to the person affected, unless they are incapable of making that decision. Encourage them to consider the impact on everyone involved in their life and also the feasibility of options based on finances.

In the end, the person requiring care must either agree with the housing choice or be deemed incapable of making the decision in order to be moved to a housing option which is safe for them. Unless they are incapacitated or deemed incapable of making their own decisions and therefore governed by a legal guardian, where they live is their decision. Sadly, that may mean that they will not be safe. And while it might not be easy to watch, we must honor their decision and do our best to see that they are as safe as possible.

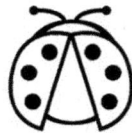

I will remember that I do not treat
a fever chart, a cancerous growth,
but a sick human being,
whose illness may affect the person's
family and economic stability.
My responsibility includes
these related problems,
if I am to care adequately for the sick.
Excerpt from the modern version of the Hippocratic Oath
written in 1964 by Louis Lasagna,
Dean of the School of Medicine at Tufts University

Chapter 6

MEDICAL CARE OPTIONS ...
matching options to your needs

Medical care facilities range from doctors' offices and small clinics to urgent care centers and large hospitals with high-tech diagnostic equipment, state-of-the-art emergency departments and trauma centers. Understanding the strength of each type of facility will help access proper treatment in a timely manner.

Each Medical Care Option Has a Purpose
There are several types of facilities for medical care, each one serving a different purpose. The choice you make in an emergency will be different from the one you make when a health issue arises but is not causing imminent danger or suffering. Following is a brief summary of each.

Immediate Medical Care Options
A ***doctor's office*** or ***medical clinic*** is the place where you *schedule an appointment* to see a specific doctor, either a primary care physician or a specialist. Typically, these visits are for annual appointments, maintenance and monitoring of an existing condition, or discussion and evaluation of a new, nonurgent symptom.

Urgent care is just that, care for medical issues that require *immediate nonemergency care*. Urgent care facilities were created to provide convenient access to treatment for *unforeseen medical needs when it is not possible to see your regular provider*. Their scope of treatment includes minor illness and injury that can be diagnosed with limited on-site equipment. They offer more availability than a medical clinic but less than the 24-hour, 365-day availability of an emergency department.

Urgent care facilities may offer services such as x-rays; lab services; and treatment of influenza, infections, allergies, wounds, and *minor* injuries. Some also offer wellness exams and immunizations. In short, these centers handle acute illnesses and injuries that would normally be treated in a physician's office and, if treated in an emergency department (ED) would cost significantly more

In some cases, an urgent care center may refer a patient to an emergency department or call paramedics to transport a patient there, for example if it seems a patient is experiencing a heart attack or requires immediate surgery.

👓👓 Mobile urgent care services offer medical providers who come to your home or work to treat urgent care needs. They will also go to a facility such as a CCRC, which is handy in eliminating the need to transport a senior for treatment.

👓👓👓 Be sure that the facility you are in is an *urgent care* and *not an emergency department*. There are now independent, free-standing emergency departments which are easily confused with urgent care facilities.

An emergency department (ED), formerly known as an emergency room, is a medical treatment facility specializing in *emergency medicine*. They provide unscheduled access for acute care of patients who often arrive via ambulance. They offer emergency medicine and extended on-site diagnostic equipment, such as MRI and CT equipment. They are available 24-hours a day, 365 days a year.

A visit to the ED is usually the result of a *major* emergent medical issue such as a heart attack or stroke requiring life-saving treatment or an injury threatening a limb. Situations that may require emergency medicine may include cases of poisoning, overdose, and the illness of babies and very young children.

Emergency departments are most often part of a hospital however, there are more offsite facilities being developed. In-hospital EDs have access to the hospital's operating rooms and surgeons.

🐞🐞 In my experience, an ED visit *always took a <u>minimum</u> of four hours* from check-in to discharge or admission to the hospital.

🐞🐞🐞 Some EDs will have a patient moved to the hospital for "observation," a status that legally can continue for three days (two midnights). Elisabeth Rosenthal, M.D., in her book "An American Sickness," explains the ramifications of this status: "Though you will be in a hospital bed, you will be considered an outpatient and be responsible for outpatient copayments and deductibles, which are generally far higher than those for an inpatient stay." She notes that Medicare will not count observation-status days toward the three inpatient days required for post-discharge coverage of a stay at a rehabilitation center or nursing home.

🐞🐞🐞 EDs are evaluated on their ability to treat major trauma before having to transfer the patient to a higher-level facility. There are five levels of trauma centers. A Level I

Trauma Center is capable of providing total care for every aspect of an injury – from prevention through rehabilitation. Separate designations are made for adult and pediatric treatment.

Following is a brief summary. This is not all inclusive and is *for conceptual comparison purposes only*. **If you have any doubt which facility to use, call them and ask when time permits, or if you are concerned that a situation may be life threatening, call 9-1-1.**

Medical office/clinic:
- For <u>scheduled</u> routine services and diagnostics
- Services provided usually within 30+ minutes
- For routine check-up or arising nonurgent symptoms
- Cost in low hundreds

👀👀 Many medical offices/clinics now offer an online patient portal providing access to a patient's important medical information, test results and future appointments. They also offer a means by which to contact the office and ask questions. These portals are invaluable in overseeing the care of another.

Urgent care:
- For <u>unscheduled</u> routine office/clinic services and **minor** conditions and injuries
- Treatment services usually provided within 1 hour,
- For diagnosis and treatment of common illnesses, including: upper respiratory infections, sinus infections and flu, as well as minor injuries such as cuts and burns.
- Cost in the 100s

Emergency department:
- For <u>unscheduled</u> **major** conditions and injuries
- Treatment services usually require a *minimum* of 4 hours
- For emergency services and treatment of life-threatening conditions and serious injuries
- Cost in the 1,000s

👀 👀 👀 **9-1-1,** while not a medical care facility, is a service that dispatches medical professionals to provide life-saving services. While an ED provides emergency medicine for life-threatening conditions and injuries, it may be necessary to call 9-1-1 for *the most immediate medical care and transportation to the ED.* There are many reasons to call 9-1-1 but a few include:
- heart attack or stroke
- loss of consciousness or head injury
- shortness of breath or difficulty breathing
- life- or limb-threatening injury or broken bones

Short to Long-Term Medical Care Options
A short-term acute care hospital (STACH) is a hospital as we usually think of one. The focus of an STACH is to diagnose and stabilize a patient after an emergency, illness, accident or surgery *within seven days.* If additional care is needed after that time period, there are a variety of transitional-care facilities – those in which the patient's strength and skills will be improved with the goal of transitioning back to home or to a long-term acute care hospital (LTACH) or facility for skilled nursing or skilled rehabilitation.

👀 👀 There are many different relationships possible between physicians and other providers (advanced nurse practitioners and PAs) and a hospital system. It is advisable to ask your provider with what STACH they are credentialed/privileged and can therefore provide treatment and services.

👀👀 *Magnet Recognition®* is the highest and most prestigious credential awarded to a healthcare organization for meeting standards for patient care, nursing excellence and innovations in nursing practice. It is designated by the American Nurses Credentialing Center. According to UC Davis Medical Center, in 2017 there were 475 Magnet hospitals accounting for about 8% of STACHs in the United States.

👀👀 If admission to an STACH is **not** an emergency and can be scheduled, such as for a nonemergency surgery, consider scheduling early in the week as STACHS are more lightly staffed on weekends and medical providers are less available. Also, if the patient will need care at home, it is more difficult to schedule those services to begin on a weekend.

👀👀 Again, if scheduling admission to an STACH is flexible, *and the STACH is a teaching facility*, consider avoiding a stay that includes July 7th. All residencies and fellowships begin and end on July 7, possibly causing a changing of the guard in medical providers.

A ***long-term acute care hospital (LTACH)*** is a transitional care hospital geared to providing long-term care for acute, ongoing conditions. An LTACH's business model requires that a patient qualify for admission, based on having one or more serious conditions that require more medical care than is offered in a skilled-nursing facility. Their focus is to provide care with the expectation that with continued care and time, the patient will return home after *an average stay of 25 days*. The bed count in an LTACH is far lower than in an STACH, often as low as a single wing of an STACH. This also means that the patient to RN and CNA ratio is significantly lower than in an STACH. Some LTACHs are stand-alone facilities and others have leased space on the floor of another hospital. The advantage to an LTACH located within an STACH is that the LTACH usually has access to the testing equipment in the STACH, eliminating the need to transport a patient from the LTACH to an STACH for testing.

For those being discharged from an STACH or an LTACH and still requiring skilled services such as medical oversight or rehabilitation therapies, **skilled nursing** is necessary. As I said previously, *skilled nursing is a service* that provides transitional care and rehabilitation to patients who require physician oversight and the services of RNs, CNAs and a social worker, as well as multidisciplinary therapy to upgrade functional ability. As transitional care, it is intended to be temporary. Because there are different reasons for staying in a SNF, they have been referred to as **convalescent care and skilled nursing**. When a patient must become a permanent resident, the SNF becomes a long-term facility sometimes referred to as a **nursing home**. Skilled-nursing services are available through a **skilled-nursing facility (SNF)**, a **skilled-rehabilitation facility (SRF)**, in a CCRC (see housing options above) and through **in-home health (IHH)** services.

For those who are not ready to return home from an STACH or LTACH, an SNF or SRF are the options. They are similar, yet different. An SNF is necessary when the medical needs of the patient are more critical than their rehabilitation needs. An SRF is designed for a short stay, during which rehabilitation requirements are greater than what is provided in an SNF, and after which the patient improves and returns home. In an SRF, therapy is done for a total of 3 hours a day, 5 days a week. The focus is to restore as much functionality as possible and to then teach patients new skills to compensate for specific lost functions.

When a patient is able to return home but still needs skilled services, whether medical, therapy or activities of daily living, in-home support services (IHSS) can be utilized. RNs and LPNs provide skilled medical services such as medication management, wound care, injections, disease management and monitoring of vitals and equipment. Licensed therapists provide physical and occupational therapies. And CNAs are available to provide assistance with ADLs such as showering. These services also include the services of a medical social worker who will work with a care plan. IHHS also provides some care supplies such as gloves and chux bed liners as needed.

🐞🐞🐞 If for any reason you are not satisfied with the care that is being provided at a medical facility, you can ask to speak with the charge RN on duty about your concerns. Some medical facilities have a patient advocate available to address urgent patient complaints and issues.

🐞🐞🐞 Many medical facilities have a *medical social worker* available to assist with a variety of services, depending on the type of facility. A social worker may be responsible for performing a complex evaluation and assessment of a patient on admission to a facility, and then may be responsible for providing assistance to the patient and their family. In most cases the social worker can help navigate insurance coverage and payment options. They may facilitate meetings between the administrative and medical teams and the patient and family members. They are usually responsible for orchestrating the patient's discharge and creating a post-discharge care plan.

🐞 🐞 🐞 🐞 Palliative and hospice care are invaluable services which are available either in-home or in many facilities. The umbrella of palliative care begins at the diagnosis of chronic, life-limiting or life-threatening illness - in short, life-altering illness – and continues through end of life. The end-of-life services offered to those no longer continuing life-extending treatments are known as hospice care. (See *Peaceful Endings*, Chapter 4 for more details.)

🐞

Selecting a Medical Care Facility

When medical care is needed, it isn't usually optional. In most cases, however, you can have input into which facility will provide the care. Whenever possible, research the options before they are needed. If you find yourself in a facility with which you are not happy, move. Most of the facilities are regulated and are required to provide you with certain services. However, some facilities tout a special service, such as memory care or Alzheimer's care, and the front-line staff is not trained to provide it. If they fail to provide the care they advertise, leave. Medical facilities are businesses and patients generate revenue. You can leave and choose another facility, whenever you want. Remember that. You never have to stand for subpar service or disrespect. *You always have a choice!*

In my experience, some facilities provided outstanding service. Sadly, some failed miserably, not only over-medicating my dad but also violating his rights. In my mom's case, the service violations were related more to providing service that was dismissive and devoid of dignity. Because my sisters and I were there to advocate for our parents, we were always able to make a better choice, but it was a learning process.

Assessing a Care Facility

When my sister and I had to evaluate LTACHs, with which we were completely unfamiliar, we had two entirely different experiences. The first location was in an old medical facility. It was dark inside, and when we approached the desk, there was no one there. In fact, we had to walk around the facility to find an employee. We were given the rundown, including that there was a doctor on call at all times. We were shown an available room that was filled with light. We asked as many questions as we could about a medical model about which we knew nothing. One of us thought to ask what happens if additional testing is needed, to which the response was that the patient had to be taken via ambulance to the hospital down the street. On our way out of the building, we encountered the family member of a patient. We asked her for input, and she informed us that her husband complained that he had to wait a very long time for a CNA to respond to the call light.

We went directly to visit a second LTACH. This visit was entirely different. The LTACH rented a wing of a hospital which offered the LTACH access to all of its diagnostic equipment. We approached and were greeted by the staff at the desk and immediately given a tour. We were told that it was a 28-bed unit, with a 1:4 ratio of RN to patient, and a 1:6 ratio of CNA to patient and had a doctor on the floor 24x7. The entire wing was light and airy and everything about it felt right.

👀 While my mom was a patient at the second LTACH we visited, she developed a blood clot in a PICC (peripherally inserted central catheter) line in her arm. Had she not been in an LTACH that had immediate access to diagnostic equipment, she might have died.

This is just an example of the value of visiting the facilities. We visited two locations offering nearly identical services, yet we came away with two entirely different feelings about them. The additional benefit in visiting both was that we then knew our alternative, if we found we needed one.

Before visiting any facility, know what you need from them, what you expect and on what you will not compromise. Many facilities are required to adhere to specific rules and regulations. If appropriate, ask about certifications and regulations and who enforces them. Make a list of questions before you visit and ask as many more questions as you possibly can. No question is stupid. If you see family of patients, ask for their permission to ask them questions and do so.

Following is a list of questions to get you started thinking about what else you might want to know. Not all questions need to be asked and for some the answer can be observed while taking a tour of the facility. Not all questions are relevant to all facilities.

- What is the out-of-pocket cost and is it affordable?
- How often is the patient seen by a doctor? When is the first visit? Is it always the same doctor?
- How soon is a care plan created?
- Is there a family meeting? If so, when and how often?
- How many patients are there?
- What is the RN to patient ratio?

- What is the CNA to patient ratio?
- What is the expected wait time for response to a call light?
- What is their restraint policy? (Is there a "no restraint" policy?)
- What is their sedation policy? (Is there a "no sedation" policy?)
- What is their philosophy on using incontinence products such as pull-ups and adult diapers?
- Are there visitation hours? Is there open visitation? Is there an overnight policy? (We stayed overnight and to be told that we could not would have been a deal breaker for us.)
- Is there an open administration policy?
- Is there exit control?
- Is there privacy?
- For those who can go outside, are there walking paths, gardens and shared space?
- If it is not an acute care facility, is there a homelike living space?
- If it is not an acute care facility, is there stimulation for the five senses?
- Do they promote independence and empowerment?
- Can the family bring in their own snacks and treats for the patient?
- Is WIFI available so that video calls can be used by family to communicate with the patient?

Many times in my life when I have had to choose an option for the provision of services, I have found it helpful to remember which way the money was flowing. In this case, the provision of medical care services, regardless of whether payment is private or through insurance, money is flowing to the facilities and the providers. You, in essence, are paying them for service rendered. If at any time you are not satisfied with the services, you have the choice to discontinue using that provider and can choose an alternative. You *always* have a choice.

Providing Comfort and Ensuring Safety in A Facility

My family's first experience in a crisis situation in a medical care facility, in this case skilled rehabilitation, did not go well for many reasons. (See *A Most Meaningful Life,* Chapter 6.) We entered the situation willing to do whatever necessary to ensure our dad's safety and comfort, but we were naïve. After an experience with our mom in an STACH, we learned what allowed us to deliver the best possible experience. Based on our experiences, we packed a suitcase with the items that would be taken with us anytime a parent was admitted to a facility. For us, our parents' comfort and safety was as important as their medical care.

What We Took

1. First, whenever possible, <u>leave all jewelry at home</u>. My grandmother had a ring stolen off her hand while in an STACH. Many facilities now photograph jewelry that the patient is wearing.

2. Second, grab the Emergency Information Book and put it in the prepacked suitcase.

3. Bring the suitcase containing:
   - Emergency Information Book (EIB) and a spiral notebook: Give a copy of the medication schedule, from the EIB, to the RN in charge.
   Write everything down, you will **not** remember it all.

- Lightweight fleece blanket: Most facility blankets are thick, heavy and rough.
- Small pillow with a distinctive pillowcase: Many of the pillows offered in facilities were large and uncomfortable.
- Nightgown: Once a hospital gown was no longer required, one of Mom's own nightgowns helped to make her feel pretty and more like herself.
- A comfortable and cozy robe
- Shoes: When possible, walking in their own rubber-soled shoes is preferable to wearing nonskid socks.
- Gym shorts: They allowed for more privacy than a gown while doing PT.
- Other clothing items: We brought old long-sleeved shirts for my dad to wear. He did not like wearing a gown and did not wear t-shirts. He was most comfortable and compliant when wearing his own clothing. The long sleeves also helped prevent Dad from pulling out his IV.
- Clean clothes for wearing home
- Plastic silverware: Many times we had to wait a very long time to get an eating utensil. We also packed straws, toothpicks and napkins.
- Condiments and other comforts: We packed those items that our parents preferred including cream, sugar, lemon juice, salt and pepper. We also included tea bags and snacks they liked.
- Nice wipes: Most facility wipes do not feel very nice and the facilities won't purchase the nice disposable wipes. We brought disposable personal wipes and offered them to the RNs and CNAs for use when cleaning our parents. We also brought Wet Ones for quick hand cleaning.

- Glasses, hearing aids, dentures and denture cleaner (Polident), and cases for their storage
- Entertainment: Give them something pleasant to pass the time, whether it is a book to read or other activity to do such as puzzle books or playing cards. My parents liked to read the newspaper, so we brought one daily. My mom read voraciously. When she began to read again, we knew that she was feeling better.
- Special supplies: My mom had a colostomy. Although the facility is supposed to provide supplies, it never happened. And what they did finally offer was not the style or brand that we needed. Therefore, we brought all of our own supplies.
- GoodNites adhesive disposable bed pads: We put these adhesive pads on the facility beds to help keep the bed clean.

4. Additional items to bring:
   - Mattress topper, sometimes called an egg crate: Many facilities require that patients be on an air mattress in order to avoid bedsores. Those mattresses caused pain for my mom, who had arthritis in her back. Most facilities did not have mattress toppers available. You will likely have to put the topper on and remake the bed yourself.
   - Bring the patient's own walker: Yes, facilities have walkers available, but it often took days to acquire one. Once my parents began to use a walker daily, we began to bring our own to a facility. It was clearly marked as our property, with masking tape with our last name on it and a big red bow on it, and we asked the facility to make a note that we had brought our own equipment.

- A Styrofoam roller for use at the end of the bed, to keep the sheets from pulling on toes and putting pressure on heels, or under knees.
- We took a couple of family photos, taken at recent family events, and had them blown up to 24" x 36". We brought them to each facility and placed them in a highly visible location, as a reminder to our parents of everyone who loved them and as a statement to the medical providers that a large family loved their patient and would be advocating for them.
- Humidifier, inexpensive and portable: Because my parents lived in a very dry climate, when a facility stay became lengthy we brought our own humidifier. It helped to keep their skin, lips, nose and throat from drying out.
- When the stay was long we brought our own source of music. It was soothing amid the frequent chaos.

What We Did

Whenever allowed and possible, we took care of our parents. They were both much more receptive to having a family member assist them than a stranger. My mom had a colostomy. We perfected the care necessary. When we entered a facility, we asked permission to continue that care. The providers really didn't want the extra work required and allowed us to use our own supplies and to do the work ourselves. It is a very personal procedure and my mom preferred that we did it. My dad had Alzheimer's and was sometimes resistant to something that a provider wanted to do to him. Again, whenever allowed, a family member would interact with dad and things went much more smoothly.

We found that in addition to what we brought to the facility, it was the simple things that made a big difference. We protected their dignity and demanded respect always. Even when the facility required they be supervised while in the bathroom, we ensured that they had privacy. Something as simple as seeing that their gowns and bedding were **always** clean and unrumpled, even if we had to do it, was invaluable in maintaining not only comfort but also a sense of dignity. Nearly always, a provider would come into the room and uncover Mom or Dad to examine them, but then fail to cover them up again. Many times one of my parents had just gotten comfortable and cozy only to be uncovered and left that way.

We pre-ordered breakfast the night before, and ordered lunch and dinner making sure that it was delivered. We made sure that things they wanted were always within their reach on their bed tray table including: a drink; Kleenex; hand wipes; lip balm and lotion; their glasses, hearing aids and dentures; and the TV control and call button. We also made sure to clean everything often and took personal laundry home to wash. We encouraged that they take a sip of their drink every 5-10 minutes. We brought photos to share, and flowers and balloons to brighten the room. Again, I believe in treating others the way I would like to be treated.

We learned a few tips that were helpful:
- Many facilities had large wheelchairs available which accommodated our dad more comfortably.
- Some facilities had toilet bars available to go over the toilet for safety.
- Tie non-skid socks to the end of the bed so that you can find them quickly when needed
- Tape a plastic spoon to each headrail closest to the part nearest the center of the bed. They can be used to keep IV tubes, etc. from getting caught on things.

- When walking in a facility and wearing a gown, wear a second gown backwards for privacy.
- Use a chip clip to hold the back of a shirt or nightgown up out of the toilet.

Because of experiences and the obvious need for patient advocacy, my family made the decision never to leave either parent alone in a medical facility. Our experiences with both parents were different. My dad had Alzheimer's, and being in an unfamiliar environment was not only disorienting but also scary. My mom had life-threatening crises that were complex. One of us was always with them to provide comfort and make critical decisions when necessary.

Finally, medical care dictates that a patient be turned or moved every two hours to avoid pressure wounds such as bed sores. That might involve shifting their weight distribution while in bed or moving them between the bed and a chair. We found that the facilities that scheduled their RNs to check on each patient every hour were good about seeing that the patients were moved. Other facilities were hit or miss on this requirement. Because a family member or one of our caregivers was always with our parents while in a facility, we saw to it that they were always moved every two hours.

👀👀 While STACHs do their best during a time of acute life-threatening illness or injury, understandably ensuring that a patient is turned is not always their top priority. After the initial crisis has been stabilized, patients are often sent to a secondary location for further care, such as LTACHs or a skilled-nursing option, and arrive with pressure wounds or skin irritations. Every facility that my parents entered did a thorough examination of them upon arrival that included

102

photographing any existing wounds or skin irritations. It was a very high priority of these facilities to treat and heal any existing wounds and to prevent new ones. They had wound care RNs treat any wounds until they were completely healed.

As soon as we could, we did the following.
- Canceled any appointments, such as hair or dental, or commitments, such as meeting with friends, of the parent in the facility.
- Let the property manager and neighbors know if no one was going to be in the home, as happened when both parents were in facilities at the same time.
- Cleaned food out of the refrigerator if both parents were not away.
- <u>Continue paying household bills.</u>
- Inventoried and reordered any medications and supplies that would be needed when the parent returned.
- Checked the mail and brought the newspaper to the facility.

Immediately prior to discharge, we made sure that the following was done:
- Groceries were purchased, especially fresh foods
- All bed and bath linens were clean
- Heat or air conditioner were adjusted to what would be comfortable
- The property manager and neighbors were notified as to when we would be returning

And throughout the process, *we thanked everyone for every helpful thing that they did* because we were genuinely grateful.

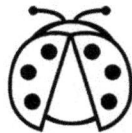

The service we render to others is really
the rent we pay for our room on this earth.
It is obvious that man is himself a traveler;
that the purpose of this world
is not "to have and to hold"
but 'to give and serve'."
Sir Wilfred T. Grenfell

Chapter 7

BUILDING YOUR CARE TEAM...
identifying the players

One of the most important tasks of the care manager is to build the care team. The care manager is the team *coach*. They are responsible for developing the team, utilizing the strengths and avoiding the weaknesses of each player, while providing constant motivation and direction based on a strategy that will result in the desired goal: dignified care and quality of life.

> Compliment people.
> Magnify their strengths,
> not their weaknesses.
> Unknown

The Team Structure
There are many players, each with their own distinct ability and responsibility, necessary for the care team to be successful: coach, quarterback, specialty players and the invaluable cheerleaders.

The following chart may be helpful in identifying the players on your team.

TEAM	name		PATIENT				
			Name Mom and Dad *dignified/compassionate care*			Helen, Jean, Joan, Grands, Greats	
			Manager/Coordinator				
			Trish				
			Patient Advocate				
			3 sisters				
			LEGAL				
			law firm name				

CAREGIVING	HEALTHCARE	INSURANCE	FINANCE	HOUSEHOLD	LEGAL	CHEER	SUPPORT
Trish	Trish					Janice, Karen	
		Barb				Susan	
Payment			Nancy	Bill payment	documents	Doris	
caregiver 1							
caregiver 1							
caregiver 1							
caregiver 1							
caregiver 1							
caregiver 1							
caregiver 1							
		Medicare, 2nd					
		long term care					
							send a gift card: coffee food
							bring food
							provide respite

The Coach and the Quarterback

Whether you are a fan, or not, a lot can be learned from America's favorite sport … football. It is a game of strategy used to achieve the ultimate goal, a win. Football is based on a specific philosophy that includes basic principles that guide the coaches in executing that strategy. While each player must follow the philosophy and adhere to the strategy, it is the responsibility of the coach to create a cohesive and cooperative team, maximizing each player's strengths. No one player is more valuable than any other, with the possible exception of the quarterback – the position that comes with decision-making responsibilities. While the coach decides what plays the team will use, the quarterback has a bird's-eye view on the field and may have to change the play in real time. So too with the care team.

As I've said, the coach's job is to oversee the entire care team, to ensure that not only are the patient's needs met but that the patient's dignity and best-possible quality of life are preserved. The coach will work with players involved in every aspect of the patient's care: medical, insurance, financial, housekeeping, legal and emotional support. The quarterback is specific to health care. They are the center of information in regard to the patient's medical treatment. Just as football quarterbacks develop relationships of trust with certain players, knowing that they can count on them to be where they are needed, the same is true for care. The health care quarterback may share some of their responsibility with trusted others, including life and death decisions, but there can always be only one quarterback. In the end, that quarterback is responsible for oversight of the medical care.

What I have said about the quarterback utilizing the input and assistance of other players, is true for all players. Trust is paramount. If a player delegates any part of their responsibility, they must know without any doubt that the delegated task will be executed on time and with accuracy. A life may depend on it.

Trust, but verify.
Ronald Reagan

In building the care team, the coach first needs to identify the care needs and those willing to share their abilities. In the beginning, the needs may be few and the quarterback may be able to serve as the patient advocate. As care needs increase, both a quarterback and a patient advocate may be required to handle other areas. The patient advocate may take on several responsibilities, or they may oversee others with specific responsibilities. Each situation is different. Ensuring that all responsibilities are covered is much more important than the team structure. In my situation, players often had multiple responsibilities, some at the detail level, others at an oversight level.

The Professionals

Medical

> The good physician treats the disease;
> the great physician treats the patient
> who has the disease.
> William Osler

There are many levels of medical providers, the experience of which it is helpful to understand.

- An *attending physician* is a physician or surgeon who has completed their residency and possibly a fellowship and is practicing their specialty.
- A *fellow* is a physician or surgeon who has completed their residency and has been accepted into a one-to-three-year fellowship program that focuses on a particular area of a specialty. Examples are fellowships in oncology after an internal medicine residency and cardiothoracic anesthesiology after anesthesiology.
- A *resident* is a physician or surgeon who has completed their medical school education and is training, under the supervision of an attending physician, for a predetermined number of years. Residencies are most often three years, however, surgical residencies are five and neurosurgery residencies last seven years.
- An *intern* is a physician or surgeon who is in the first year of their residency. Some specialties require a separate year of internship before beginning a residency.

- Physician Assistant (PA)
- Advanced Practice Registered Nurse
  - Nurse Practitioner
  - Certified Nurse-Midwife
  - Certified Registered Nurse Anesthetists
  - Clinical Nurse Specialists
- Registered Nurse

		PATIENT			
		patient name			patient support
		dignified/compassionate care			family/close friends
Date:	xx/xx/xx	Attending Physician			
Location:	*xxx hospital*	Specialty		*hospitalist, specialist*	
		Name			
		Fellows			
		Residents			
		Interns			

	Specialist	Specialist	Specialist	Specialist
Specialty				
Name				
Fellows				
Residents				
Interns				
Charge RNs				
RNs				
CNAs				
Phlebotomists				

Nonmedical

Enlisting the assistance of any professionals who have worked with the patient in the following areas is invaluable.

- Lawyers (See *Peaceful Endings*, Chapter 2, Understanding Estate Planning.)
- Financial Planners
- Accountants
- Insurance Agents and Companies

In some situations, a social worker may be available to assist with identifying options and making decisions. Many hospitals and care facilities have a social worker on staff, and each county has a senior resource and services department.

Caregivers

Caregivers come in many forms, some are professionals, such as Certified Nurse Assistants (CNAs) and Home Health Aides (HHAs), and others are unskilled caregivers including family or friend volunteers. In any case, caregivers provide care in the form of everything from companionship to assistance with activities of daily living (ADLs). (See Chapter 8.)

Family and friends

Let me start by saying two things:

1. The family's role is to provide comfort and to protect, respect and preserve dignity. They are to act as another pair of eyes overseeing medical and non-medical care. Family is also the keeper of the patient's history, knowing not only the patient's baseline and their past history but also their most current history.

2. Children do not belong on the care team. Do not ask them to provide care or to translate for someone who speaks a language different from the one being used to convey information. Just don't.

   Children, particularly grandchildren and great-grandchildren, are a source of joy to their grandparents and great-grandparents. While they are not technically a part of the care team, their contribution is invaluable. The same is true of family pets.

Once the care needs have been identified, it is a matter of matching those needs to the abilities of others. Previously, I discussed that responsibility is one's response to their ability. Everyone has abilities, limitations and emotional triggers. Most often the real challenge is to motivate people to offer their abilities. Some will not be able to respond with an offer of active help for a variety of reasons: inability, unwillingness, logistics, family commitments and financial constraints, to name a few. But there is always something they can do to be supportive. It is the job of the coach to determine how best to use each person's abilities to meet the needs of the person requiring care.

> A person's most useful asset is not
> a head full of knowledge,
> but a heart full of love,
> an ear ready to listen and
> a hand willing to help.
> Unknown

Involving family and friends in care can be a double-edged sword. In Chapter 1 of *Peaceful Endings,* I discussed the dynamics of families and the value of rising above childhood roles and wounds. Forgiving and forgetting the past is the only way families can work together to provide the best care possible. There should be a clear understanding that all actions must be in the patient's greatest interest, and nothing else will be tolerated.

Crisis, whether the short sprint or the marathon, causes some family members to step into what I call "the trench," the place of daily involvement and active participation in care and life decisions. The trench is not for everybody, and each family member makes their own decision, one with which they will have to live. Those who cannot step into the trench can best contribute by providing support for those who do.

Sadly, we've all heard the phrase, "every family has one," one being a member who makes excuses, does not participate, is not supportive or tries to manage from a distance. While their intention might be to help, it is best for those who are at a distance to understand that those in the center are doing their best. That said, I know that some days my best didn't look like it. I was exhausted and frustrated, trying to find answers and solutions without enough information, and some days I felt like I had just plain failed. Regardless, it was still the best that I had to offer on that particular day. I was always doing my best.

In all situations, various family members will participate at different levels. It can be helpful to provide a time for every family member to express their feelings about the situation. Each feeling should be heard with respect and without judgment whether or not there is agreement with it. This may release some of the emotion connected to the care situation and clear the air for more open communication. Each person has made their decision about offering their abilities based on factors others may or may not understand, and each person has to live with their decisions.

I cannot speak enough about the differences in experience for those who are "in the trench" and those who are not. The trench is the place closest to the patient, at the epicenter of the care situation, the place that can feel a bit like being in a personal war zone defending dignified and compassionate care and upholding the rights of the patient. It is not better or worse, more valuable or less, to be in the trench. It is merely significantly different. Having spoken to many families who have provided care, there has been a common experience where a family member who is not in the trench will arrive, usually from out of town, to "fix" all that they perceive is being done wrong by those in the trench. Everyone, including those not in the trench, is entitled to an opinion and *to offer constructive criticism when delivered with viable alternatives*. No one has the right to criticize without offering to participate in the solution.

> If you aren't in the arena
> also getting your ass kicked,
> I'm not interested in your feedback.
> Brene Brown

It's a little like providing commentary from the safety of your home to someone on the front lines of war. Those at home are entitled to their opinions, but they truly do not understand the reality of the situation nor have they made themselves available to participate in or positively impact it.

> There were the visits from my brother
> when he "took over the worry"
> so that I could … just live.
> Marky Olson, *Caregiving for Your Elderly Parents*

Those observing from a distance have a special responsibility: to be supportive of those at the epicenter. That can come in many forms. (See Postscript.) They may or may not be willing or able to provide respite for those that are more involved, but when they can it is immensely helpful and appreciated.

Friends often want to help, offering everything from occasional visits and respite to entrenching themselves in a care schedule. While good intentioned, friends add another dynamic for the care manager. With rare exception and only when necessary, or in the absence of family, is it advisable for friends be part of a care team. Providing care is often a difficult time for families, sometimes requiring siblings to work in an emotional pressure cooker, which is at best highly personal. Again, it is advisable to use caution when relying on friends for help, and possibly best to ask only for occasional, very specific, assistance and emergency coverage only. Friends may be best utilized in providing **you** with support in your life.

The Support Team
Every team needs cheerleaders. They are the backbone of the support team: those who cheer for the often tired and sometimes frustrated and defeated care team members. Support comes in many forms, from providing for a specific need of the patient to assisting a care team member with their personal life, and is equally important to the care team as the care team is to the patient. (See the Postscript.)

The job of the support team is not only important but sometimes challenging. Those you entrust to listen to the frustration and disappointment of a care team member provide an invaluable outlet. That outlet, however, can sometimes be a bit depressing and heavy, as you are in essence asking the support person to carry some of your emotional load at times. It is important to remember that if you are going to ask a support person to carry, if only by listening, some of the negative energy of your experience, it is then important to share some of the positive experiences.

114

Even in most dire situations, there will be levity, laughter or a surprise jewel of a moment. Remember to share those as well as the heaviness of the other experiences.

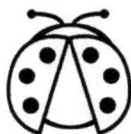

There are only four kinds
of people in the world –
those who have been caregivers,
those who are currently caregivers
those who will be caregivers
and those who will need caregivers.
Rosalynn Carter

Chapter 8

FINDING CAREGIVERS ...
finding the right fit

The conversation about bringing hired caregivers into a home is delicate. It can threaten the idea of a person's independence and competence, and often sparks worry about theft and worse. My mom assisted with the care of my grandparents but lived 1,000 miles away. My grandparents were vulnerable, as my grandmother was not mobile without assistance, and my grandfather had diminished sight and hearing. Sadly, my grandparents did experience theft. My mom did the best that she could to provide care until she was able to move my grandparents into her home where she could provide and supervise additional care.

When I moved to Denver, my mom had already hired someone to come into their home to assist with light chores and to provide respite for mom's oversight of dad for a few hours, three days a week. Once Dad had his first medical crisis, during which my family oversaw his care 24x7, and knowing that my parents wanted to stay in their home until their final day, my sisters and I approached Mom about bringing in a skilled caregiver to help with Dad. She was reluctant but understood that we could not physically or emotionally continue the 24x7 care that we had been providing. I assured Mom that I would oversee the hiring of caregivers, and that I would replace them if I had any doubt about their skill or honesty. I will always be grateful that Mom trusted my sisters and me, and agreed to the skilled caregivers. We all knew that this marked the beginning of continual care.

If you are ready to hire skilled caregivers, then you likely have completed the following "prerequisites." You: accepted a new responsibility to manage the care of another (see Chapter 1), understand the need for constant patient advocacy (see Chapter 2), have reviewed the details of managing care (see Chapter 3), have identified the care needs (see Chapter 4) and, based on those care needs, you have built your team (see Chapter 7). Now it is time to prepare to provide care.

The best way to find yourself
is to lose yourself in the service of others.
Mahatma Gandhi

You may be providing care in a home or maybe in a facility. Even if you have chosen a facility, your situation may require additional care. Facilities cannot oversee each patient constantly, and our situation required that. We needed to provide 24x7 oversight, requiring an awake overnight caregiver.

Once you fully know your needs, both care and scheduling, your first step may be to identify caregivers. Finding caregivers is based on knowing the options, making conscious informed choices based on your needs and realistically fitting the puzzle pieces together based on all of your variables.

That horrifying moment when
you're looking for an adult but
you realize that you are an adult.
So you look around for an older adult,
an adultier adult adulting,
someone better at it than you.
Unknown

🐞🐞🐞🐞 I want to be clear that the *use of the term hiring in this book does not imply employment* but rather is used to reference the process of finding a caregiver to provide care. Whether a caregiver is considered an employee is determined by the source of the caregiver, the business relationship between the caregiver and patient and state laws. In no way am I providing information or advice on that status.

🐞

Nonmedical Caregivers

The information below addresses only *nonmedical care*. Medical care is detailed in Chapter 6. Nonmedical care is available from nonskilled and skilled caregivers, those who have completed formal training and certification and/or licensing. Caregivers can be hired in a variety of ways. There are pros and cons to each alternative. It may come down to a combination of financial resources and how much risk you're willing to assume.

🐞🐞 Medical insurance typically does not cover nonmedical caregivers. Medicare does not cover nonmedical caregivers. Long-term care insurance often covers caregivers but requires that they be skilled and have credentials, such as a CNA or HHA certification.

There are two types of nonmedical caregivers:
1. *Unskilled caregivers* have not been trained and are not certified or licensed to assist with ADLs. They can however, provide companionship, respite and may be able to assist with some of the IADLs such as managing money, cooking, housekeeping, shopping or errands, leisure activities and transportation.

2. ***Skilled caregivers*** have been trained to assist with ADLs. *They may or may not be certified or licensed.* They are skilled in providing assistance with the following activities:
   o Bathing/showering
   o Personal hygiene and grooming (brushing/combing hair, oral care)
   o Dressing
   o Toilet hygiene (getting on/off, cleaning oneself), including continence
   o Functional mobility or transferring (walking, getting into and out of a bed or chair
   o Self-feeding

Caregiver services are typically available for an hourly rate or for a 24-hour rate. Some services offer a short shift for which rates are slightly lower. Some caregivers offer live-in rates, meaning they literally live with the patient 24x7. Other caregivers will offer 24-hour shifts, requiring a sleeping space in the location of the patient but returning to their own home when they are off shift.

Before contacting an agency, registry or independent caregiver, be sure to know exactly what your needs and requirements are and whether you require unskilled or skilled caregivers and whether they need to be certified or licensed. This is particularly important if you will be working with independent caregivers whom you want covered by long-term care insurance.

Prices listed below are for <u>relative comparison</u>. Check with local home-care agencies, home-care registries and independent caregivers for current pricing.

Considerations for Selecting a Source for Caregivers

There are many things that must be considered in deciding where to source your caregivers.

There are many tasks that must be done when working with caregivers. If you hire through an agency or registry, that organization will probably handle these functions. Home-care agencies and registries charge a premium for the additional services that they provide. If you hire an independent caregiver, someone must perform these tasks. While working with independent caregivers may cost up to 40% less, you must consider whether you want the responsibilities.

The projected duration of care needed may be a factor. If it is short term, you may want to pay a business to handle the administrative requirements. For a long duration of care, you may be willing to be responsible for the administrative components in trade for the cost savings. That may be dependent on whether you have the time, the skill and the desire to handle the following responsibilities or ensure that all necessary items are in place. If not, you may choose to hire someone to execute the tasks.

- Identifying and screening the candidates based on your needs and their skills and experience. It also requires a background check and checking all of their references.
  Be aware of the information that is included in a specific background check.
- Training requires walking the caregiver through your environment and requirements and also should be documented for future reference.

121

- <u>Determining duties</u> is based on your needs and the ability of each caregiver to meet them.
- <u>Supervising</u> caregivers is necessary.
- <u>Scheduling</u> especially when multiple caregivers are involved. Remember to schedule caregiver time off and vacations.
- <u>Backup care</u> is necessary to cover caregiver absences due to illness as well as time off that is scheduled in advance..
- <u>Patient's safety</u> is always paramount and must be monitored. Putting the patient at risk should result in termination.

  👀👀 We had **safety words**. The use of a specific pre-determined word indicated that my parents needed one of us to come over as soon as possible. The use of another word indicated that we were to call 911 immediately. We also frequently dropped in unexpectedly.
- <u>Behavior issues, inability to provide service and complaints</u> must be addressed and appropriate discipline enforced.
- <u>Termination of services</u> may be necessary. Services are provided "at will" and can be terminated at any time and for any reason including that the caregiver and client are not a "good fit." It may be a philosophical difference or a personality clash. If a fit is not good for the client, it is likely not good for the caregiver either.
- <u>Insurance</u> - Caregivers should be bonded and/or insured either through an agency or registry or independently.

  👀👀 Agencies and some registries are bonded and/or insured and provide worker's compensation. Independent caregivers should be bonded or insured for liability and carry worker's compensation insurance, although many do not. Homeowners should check with their insurance agent to be sure that they are protected from liability in the event that a caregiver is injured while working in their home. Generally, homeowners are covered by homeowners' insurance and can't be sued as long as the home is safe from foreseeable safety risks. Discuss with your insurance agent whether you want to purchase an additional umbrella policy.

- <u>Payment</u> - Hours/shifts and payment must be tracked in an accurate, organized manner. Depending on the situation, working with an independent caregiver may require withholding and payment of taxes.

  🐞🐞 Check with an accountant regarding the laws in your state.

- <u>Cost</u> varies depending on your caregiver source.

Caregiver sources include home-care agencies, home-care registries and independent caregivers.

Home-Care Agencies

A home-care agency is licensed and regulated by the state. It hires caregivers, checks their backgrounds and references, provides training, handles their payment and covers them under worker's compensation. The caregivers are employees of the agency. Therefore, the fee for the caregivers includes the expense for those services, as well as the administrative costs of the business which include licensing and insurance or bonding. While trained and tested by the agency and therefore considered skilled, *the caregivers may or may not be certified.* Agencies will provide a replacement if the regularly scheduled caregiver will be absent from work, however the replacement may be unfamiliar to the patient and with the environment. It is important to meet a caregiver prior to the first day of service to be sure they are a good fit with the patient.

Prices may be $22-$26/hour, with a 3-hour minimum, or $225-$300 for a 24-hour shift. The caregiver may be *compensated $10/hour or $110 for a 24-hour shift, with the agency keeping the significant portion of the fee.*

Home-Care Registries

A home-care registry is a referral service for caregivers. They provide families with a list of possible candidates, but do not employ the caregivers. Because they have less overhead than an agency, their fees are less than an agency but more than an independent caregiver. Registries have access to backup caregivers in the event that your regularly scheduled caregiver is absent. As with an agency, replacement caregivers may be unfamiliar to the patient and with the environment. It is important to meet a caregiver prior to the first day of service to be sure they are a good fit with the patient. A registry charges a finder's fee that is paid to the registry, in addition to the fee that is paid directly to the caregiver. As with the agency, the entire fee is paid for the duration of the services.

Prices may be $25/day for the registry (paid until services are terminated) and $18/hour or $180 for a 24-hour shift. The caregiver receives the entire $18/hour or $180 for the 24-hour shift.

Independent Caregivers

Independent caregivers may also be employed by an agency and/or listed on a registry, but also offer their services independently. Being an employee of an agency or listed on a registry may only provide the caregiver with part-time work, allowing them to find additional work independently. Be aware that any benefits offered for that caregiver when contracted through an agency or registry are not available when working with the caregiver independently.

In short, working with independent caregivers is significantly less expensive than through an agency or registry, however, the list of tasks above is all your responsibility. You are on your own.

Prices may be $15/hour or $180 for a 24-hour shift. The caregiver receives the entire hourly or 24-hour shift rate.

Working with Independent Caregivers

If you choose to work with independent caregivers you will be responsible for the administrative tasks involved.

Identifying and screening

Independent caregivers can be found in a variety of ways, including on websites, as well as by word of mouth. Care.com connects clients with caregivers and is an excellent place to start your search. The website requires you to create a free account to post a job, preview responses and browse caregivers near you. Once you want to use their screening tools and communicate with caregivers, you can choose to pay a subscription fee. This fee allows you to view full profiles, reviews, references, and contact information. Background checks can be conducted for an additional fee, although you may want to do your own background check depending on what information you want and the cost. I *do not* recommend using craigslist.org to find caregivers, as it does not provide any of the services that care.com does. Caregivers have a sort of network where they have come to know each other and refer each other as well. Once you have broken into that network, it is easier to find them.

The process of identifying and screening a caregiver might be:
1. Write and place an ad. Be as specific and clear as possible. (See example in next section.)

2. When you get a response, Google the person's name. If the person has a common name, you may have to put your state prior to the name. If you do not find anything of concern, contact the person.
3. Set up an in-person interview, requiring a resume, references, certificates, Social Security card and driver's license or state id. Discuss the job requirements, caregiver agreement, start date and trial period, scheduling, compensation and pay cycle. Make sure they know that they are responsible for having their own liability and disability insurance.
4. You may want to Google the person's name again based on any new information from the interview, such as where they lived previously.
5. Check the caregiver's references, only if you are interested in the candidate.
6. Run a background check and verify any other information desired, such as certifications. Again, do this only if you are interested in the candidate and their references were good, as there may be expense involved in this process.

It is essential that a background check be run and that all references be checked prior to working with a new caregiver. I checked references for a caregiver that presented very well, only to find out what had happened on a previous job. I cannot imagine that the person actually gave me her previous employer as a reference. It was shocking and we did not hire the caregiver.

👀 When calling a business for a reference check, you may be limited by law in what they can share with you. Sometimes the only questions they can answer are whether the person had worked at the business and if the business would rehire them.

In addition to doing a background check and checking references, consider whether you want to check the following:

- Driving record
  Driving records can be obtained from the state DMV.
- Drug screening
  Contact a LabCorp or Quest Diagnostics in your area to find out how to arrange for a drug test.
- Sex offender database
  The Dru Sjodin National Sex Offender Public website (www.nsopw.gov) is provided by the U.S. Department of Justice to facilitate a free nationwide search for sex offenders. Searches can be done by name or location.
- Healthcare training credentials
  To verify CNA certification, Google the name of your state followed by "CNA certification verification."

The following websites may be helpful in doing a background check. Google: "your state" followed by "Bureau of Investigation." Once on the website, you may have to search on "public" or "Internet" followed by "background check" or "records check". The same can be done with the Federal Bureau of Investigation. Another resource is c3Intelligence (www.c3intelligence.com), a reasonably priced service that provides a search for national and county criminal records and national sex offenders. Finally, you can Google: "how to do a background check."

If your care needs are long term, identifying and screening will likely be ongoing. In 18 months my family worked with 17 caregivers. There were several reasons we went through so many to end up with a team of seven. Caregiving is a tough job, in particular for those who work 24-hour shifts. Some caregivers needed to move on to different shifts and we could not offer them another shift. We wished them well on their way, wrote them outstanding letters of recommendation and will always be grateful for their service. One caregiver left to attend college, another we knew was temporary, a couple had marginal skills, one was rude to my parents, another was just plain lazy, and another was, well I don't know what to say about that.

Providing training
Training is necessary to introduce the caregiver to the patient, and if it is in-home care , to the environment. We did training for each of our caregivers. We created a training script to follow to be sure to cover everything that was important to us and dedicated at least one full shift to be present and work with them. In addition, training may be needed for any task unfamiliar to the caregiver that you want your caregiver to do.

Determining duties
Clarification of each caregiver's duties is important, especially if there are multiple caregivers. It ensures that all needs are met and that oversight or duplication do not happen. Also agencies have strict rules on what tasks can be performed by a caregiver. Many do not allow their caregivers to drive to appointments, do errands or attend social activities with the client. Independent caregivers are more flexible in what they can and will do.

Supervision
Regardless of whether a caregiver has been contracted through an agency and is overseen by someone at that agency, supervision is necessary. You need to ensure that the

responsibilities are being met and that the caregiver is a good fit with the patient. We had one in-home health RN who did a good job, but with whom Mom was not comfortable. Once she expressed her feelings, we requested a different RN, stating that it was just "not a good fit."

Long-distance supervising is difficult, but it is not impossible. Technology offers video chatting and video monitoring, and there are products that assist with monitoring care long distance. (See Chapter 11, *Assistance, Safety, Comfort and Convenience*, Safety, Monitoring.)

Scheduling
Scheduling is an important responsibility and can be a big task if there are multiple caregivers involved. We needed care for two parents. Initially we had two 24-hour caregivers, one working three days and the other working the remaining four. Later we added a 12-hour shift shared by two caregivers during the week. And even later we added a 12-hour awake night shift shared by two caregivers. Including one sister and me, there were nine caregivers scheduled in a given week. Our caregivers were incredibly dedicated and requested extremely little time off. In fact, they began to cover each other's absences. When we offered them holidays off, they were reluctant because they had never had that option. We were able to offer it to them because family was always with my parents on the holidays.

Backup care
Even with the best caregivers, unexpected absences occur. We had requested that our caregivers *not* come in to work if they were not well. I received a call at 6:30 a.m. from a caregiver who was not well. I covered that shift.

Behavior issues, inability to provide service and complaints
Working with anyone can present challenges. Working with caregivers may present unusual challenges, because the situation is already stressful and in-home scenarios are more personal and complicated. Behavioral and service issues and complaints must be addressed.

Termination
Termination of services may be necessary. It's not pleasant but believe me, if a caregiver disrespects someone you love, you will find out how easy it can be. One of my sisters had a friend who had experience with caregivers. She provided us with guidance in regard to writing an ad and identifying duties. Her last piece of advice was to "hire them and fire them." I heard that advice but thought it was a bit harsh. By the time we had to terminate service with a few caregivers, I understood. Hire them, and if it's not working out, fire them. It's not personal, it's business. And the phrase, "it's not a good fit" is invaluable.

Insurance
As I said before, caregivers should be bonded and/or insured either through an agency or registry or independently. That includes liability insurance and worker's compensation.

Payment
Payment goes hand in hand with scheduling. It requires the tracking of hours/shifts worked. This gets a bit complicated when caregivers change shifts or are absent. We tracked the weekly schedule and required caregivers to log their hours. When a change in the schedule was made, it was recorded on a calendar so that everyone was aware of who would be working the shift.

🐞 We found that several caregivers did not have checking accounts and were therefore being charged a significant sum to cash their checks. We found a bank that would not charge the caregivers to cash their checks as long as they cashed them at the bank on which the check was written. It was a small inconvenience for us to open a new account, but a big benefit to the caregivers.

🐞

Sample Caregiver Ad
Below is a sample ad for a caregiver:

Please note the applicant requirements below before responding. Thank you.

What we are looking for:
Two caregivers to split a 24/7 schedule, possibly Sunday 9 a.m. - Thursday 9 a.m. and Thursday 9 a.m. - Sunday 9 a.m. (24 hour shifts), to help care for our father. Days/times are negotiable.

About the client:
He is a kind and a gentle man of 91 years with Alzheimer's. He may or may not remember your name but he is likely to say "thank you" and tell you he loves you. He has always loved to tease and be a bit silly. Like any of us, he tends to get upset when you do something that physically hurts him or is really thoughtless. Walking is difficult as he has a bad hip and bad knee. He is supposed to use a walker but often forgets.

He lives with his wife of 68 years and all of his family lives nearby, mostly in the Denver metro area, and drop by frequently. We have helped provide 24/7 oversight for him for the past several years.

What is needed:
Constant oversight is needed for safety and some assistance (verbal queuing and supervision) with the activities of daily living, which could include dressing, bathroom assistance (currently with grooming, toileting and possibly showering in the future), and managing medications. Additional duties to include meal prep, laundry, light housekeeping and some grocery shopping.

Applicant requirements:
- MUST be a CNA or Home Health Aide, licensed/certified in Colorado,
- have experience with dementia, preferably Alzheimer's,
- have your own transportation,
- be a nonsmoker,
- provide resume, proof of license/certifications, references, background check, and
- must be willing to provide Social Security number if hired.

LOCATION: SE Denver

Comparing Caregiver Sources
The following chart shows a summary of who is responsible for each of the specific tasks required when working with caregivers.

| Tasks | Agency | Registry | Independent | |
			You	Caregiver
Identifying and screening	Y	Y	Y	
Reference checks	Y	Y	Y	
Background Checks, etc.	Y	Y	N	
Bonding and Insurance	Y	Y	homeowners +/or umbrella	liability and worker's comp
Licensing	* Y	* Y	verify	Y
Training	Skills	Skills	special skills	Skills
Determining Duties	** Y	** Y	YYY	
Match caregivers to families	Y	Y	Y	
Supervising	*** Y	*** Y	YYY	
Scheduling	Y	N	YYY	
Patient's safety	Y	N	YYY	
Payment	Y	N	Y	
Taxes, *if required*	Y	N	Y	
Behavior issues and complaints	Y	N	Y	
Termination	Y	Y	Y	
Back-up care	Y	Y	Y	
Your time off/vacations	N	N	Y	
Provide Nursing Care	N	N		N unless RN
EXAMPLE, **relative prices**, shown as paid/caregiver's paid				
Daily Upcharge		25/0		
Hourly	22/10	18/18	15/15	
24-hours	225/110	180	180/180	

NOTE: "Y" indicates that **most** agencies and registries are responsbile for that task. Always verify that they do.

"* Y" = Licensing is for the agency or registry and the caregivers are covered under the oragnization. It does not indicate that the caregiver is licensed as in individual.

"** Y" = The agency or registry helps to identify duties and specific skills needed. You identify your needs and ultimately the duties requied..

"*** Y" = Agencies and registries don't really uspervise the day-to-day work of a caregiver. They drop in to see how things are going. You, or someone you trust, will have to supervise the caregivers.

"YYY" = Even if an agency or registry is involved with the task, you will be instrumental in its execution.

133

Other Considerations Regarding All Caregivers

Each item in this entire section gets 🐞🐞🐞 for importance.

1. CNA is often used to describe nonmedical caregivers. Certified CNAs have attended and passed training, and have passed a *state certification test*. Some skilled caregivers have taken and passed the training but have failed or did not take the state test. They are skilled caregivers but not CNAs, as the "C" stands for certified. To verify CNA certification, Google the name of your state followed by "CNA certification verification." CNA certification is state specific. Some states offer reciprocity through which a certification can be transferred to the state. Others require that a CNA certify by taking the test in the new state.

    🐞🐞 Home-health aides (HHAs) have similar but different training and may or may not be certified. An HHA may be an option for your situation.

    🐞🐞 I use the term caregiver loosely because we had many levels of nonmedical caregivers: unskilled, skilled and certified. I use the term caregiver to refer to the job of providing care as opposed to referring to a skill level.

2. Most states require that a caregiver have medication administration training before administering medications to a client. Additional training and certification through a qualified medication administration curriculum (QMAP) may be necessary. QMAP certification verification can be found by Googling "QMAP verification."

134

3. While not necessarily required to provide care, many caregivers have additional certifications such as for Cardio-Pulmonary Resuscitation (CPR) and first aid, and in the use of an automatic external defibrillator (AED).

4. Patient safety is paramount. I promised my parents that I would keep them safe. For me, that included safe from injury, harm, fear, disrespect and theft. Safety was our top priority, and that required supervision and monitoring. A safety violation was cause for termination of service. In one instance, I began to think that we should put cameras in my parents' home. I then realized that if I doubted someone's honesty enough to install cameras to watch them, I did not trust them and therefore had to terminate their services. As stated above, we used safety words as a means to know if a parent did not feel safe and was in need of immediate help.

5. Bonding is *conceptually similar* to insuring, yet far less favorable for the client. For example, if an agency or caregiver is *insured* and a client claims theft by the caregiver, the client reports the theft and the claim ultimately will be paid by the insurer that covers the caregiver. If the agency or caregiver is *bonded* and there is a claim of theft, <u>the bonding company does not have to reimburse the client until the theft has been validated in a court of law. This requires the client to have the caregiver arrested, charged and convicted in a criminal court before the bond is paid.</u>

6. Caregivers provided by agencies and registries *may or may not be state certified*. Agencies train and test, and therefore caregivers may be covered by long-term care

insurance under the agency licensing. A registry does not provide training and has accepted the caregiver based on their experience. When working for an agency or referred by a registry, the caregivers are not required to be state certified in order to be covered by long-term care insurance. If a caregiver employed by an agency or referred by a registry is later employed independently, the decision as to whether they will be covered by long-term care insurance will be based on whether they are state certified.

7. Any caregiver that you work with through an agency or registry cannot be hired independently for a period of usually six months to a year, depending on their contract, after you terminate their caregiving services.

🐞🐞 Additional information on caregiver sources can be found on www.caring.com and by Googling "home care agency," "home care registry" or "independent caregivers."

Benefits of the 24-Hour Shift
24-hour shifts are paid at less than an hourly rate. While there is clearly a monetary benefit to the patient, there is value added for the caregiver. My family created and identified additional benefits to the caregiver. This list is based on what we were willing to offer our caregivers. Also, keep in mind that a 24-hour caregiver is provided with a private space in which to sleep for a minimum of 8 hours.

9 Benefits of a 24-Hour Shift
1.) Private bedroom, sheets and towels provided, TV and Internet in the bedroom as well as access to Netflix

2.) Meals/drinks provided, three meals a day and snacks

3.) At times another person, either a family member or another shift caregiver on-site to do some tasks and to assist when needed

4.) Either an additional rest time during the day or assistance at night if the patient requires assistance more than two times during the night

5.) Not paying for their own utilities at home while working

6.) Can do their laundry while they are working

7.) Have access to TV, Internet and Netflix during down time

8.) Less wear and tear on their car and reduced gas costs by not commuting daily

9.) Not coming and going in the dark and snow to be home nine hours, sleep and return

Working with caregivers will likely be evolutionary, beginning with one set of needs and ending with full care. Your situation may initially be as simple as needing a caregiver to provide companionship, respite and/or minimal assistance with an ADL, such as showering. It may also be as complex as scheduling several caregivers throughout the week to provide 24x7 assistance with all ADLs. The following chapter addresses actually working with caregivers.

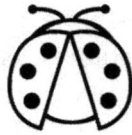

Caregivers are often the casualties,
the hidden victims.
No one sees the sacrifices they make.
Judith L. London

Chapter 9

PROVIDING CARE ...

the art of finesse

Two responsibilities are paramount in the caregiver's role - - to ensure the client's safety and to preserve the client's dignity. Caregiving requires a delicacy in execution, subtlety in handling difficult or sensitive situations, tact, diplomacy, elegant skill and artful management. Simply put, it requires finesse.

My family's situation was evolutionary, starting with one part-time, non-skilled caregiver and ending with a team of nine skilled caregivers providing full-time care for both parents. Most situations will not be as complex, but ours is a good example because it covers so many challenges. In 2011, my parents began the process of bringing caregivers into their home. It started with one part-time, nonskilled caregiver assisting with household tasks and overseeing my dad's safety when my mom went out. The caregiver worked 4 hours a day, three days a week for several months. By fall of 2012, two skilled caregivers (certified CNAs) shared a 24x7 shift allowing one caregiver to be present at all times, including overnight. These caregivers were primarily assisting my dad with ADLs, overseeing his safety, preparing meals and occasionally assisting my mom. In the spring of 2013, we added a 12-hour skilled caregiver (certified CNAs) day shift to care for my mom while she was recovering from a medical crisis. By fall 2013, an additional 12-hour shift was added requiring that the skilled caregiver be awake to oversee my dad. At that point, we had nine caregivers, including one sister and me, on the weekly schedule. As I said, our situation was unusually complex as we needed full-time care for both parents. We created many forms and documents, such as daily log sheets and newsletters, to help manage our parents' care and to create a cohesive care team. You may not need all of the information that follows, but you are likely to need some of it. Some of this information may prompt you to think about issues that may need to be addressed in the future.

Working with Caregivers

Caregivers are very special people. They are willing to provide care that family often cannot or will not. It is often a challenging job, but one which returns great rewards.

Skilled caregivers are trained to assist with all of the ADLs, each of which can present challenges depending on the client's ability to assist with the task. For example, making a bed may require that it be done with the client in the bed. Other tasks such as assisting with a bath and washing someone's hair or changing an undergarment may have to be done in bed as well. Assisting with mobility may involve the proper use of a gait belt or the managing of a walker or wheelchair. Transferring a person from one location to another, from a bed to a chair or into and out of a car, for example, can be difficult depending on the ability of the person to bear weight and pivot. And taking vitals can present its own challenges. Clearly skilled caregivers are indeed skilled, and they have been hired based on their skill.

The greatest gift you can give someone
is your time.
Because when you give your time,
you are giving a portion of your life
that you will never get back.
Unknown

Caregivers enter the lives of a client when they most need help. Too often, caregivers work with clients who have no family nearby or no one to help them, and the caregiver provides not only care but also companionship and compassion. In most cases the caregiver is working their shift alone.

Sometimes care is provided in a private home, where family members have invited the caregivers in to tend to the family's most precious members, and the caregivers become part of the family. That was our situation. When we started having caregivers, my mom was not only in the home and cognitively well, she was also medically well. The caregivers, each working a one-person shift, had to do their job with Mom's constant oversight. As the care team grew, many of our caregivers had to learn how to work within a team, not only providing dignified care but also being respectful of each other and communicating to provide consistent care.

Be a reflection
of what you'd like to see in others.
if you want love, give love.
If you want honesty, give honesty.
If you want respect, give respect.
You get in return, what you give.
Unknown

We understood that our family had put our trust in the caregivers to care for, protect and keep safe the most important people in our lives, our parents. We welcomed the caregivers, made them feel at home and treated them well. In short, we cared for our caregivers. We bought them birthday and Christmas gifts, occasionally left a holiday cookie or treat in their communication center folder and celebrated their joys while supporting their challenges. We provided the caregivers with house keys; bought the coffee and snacks they enjoyed; bought magazines and puzzle books; and registered for Netflix for their use.

We truly appreciated their help and thanked them for even the smallest thing. Our caregivers came to love our parents as our parents loved them, and they brought my parents things they thought they would enjoy or would be helpful, as well as little surprises or treats. Some of them became more than family, they became friends. And in return, the caregivers cared not only for our parents but also for my sisters and me.

> Being told you're appreciated
> is one of the simplest and most uplifting things
> you can hear.
> Sue Fitzmaurice

Part of providing the best care possible for our parents required caring for our caregivers by being organized, being clear about expectations and responsibilities, having information easily accessible to them and providing them with the best tools and supplies needed to do their job. We also provided training when necessary. Some caregivers were more skilled at some tasks than others, and being aware of that allowed us to help each caregiver be successful, resulting in job satisfaction. Each caregiver arrived with valuable experience, from which we knew we could learn and benefit. We encouraged our caregivers to offer suggestions and ideas for improvement, as well as to ask questions. In many situations, it was a caregiver's idea or question that prompted us to re-evaluate a process and make positive changes. We created a cohesive team of caregivers, who then began to work together as a unit and earned our trust.

The first three things we created were the Caregiver Agreements and Responsibilities, Daily Objectives and Requirements for Each Shift and The Caregiver Book. These documents were very detailed, and while some of it may even seem unnecessary, we found that things went most smoothly when we documented our needs and made it easily available for future reference. We also found that our caregivers thrived on the information. The clearer and more detailed we were, the more empowered they were to be successful.

Following are some of the *documents we created to provide clarity as well as the tools that we used to assist our caregivers.* Again, this is just what my family did to work with caregivers. I am providing it as *an example from which you can customize your own tools.*

🐞🐞 Examples of the documents that my family used with our caregivers are posted on and can be downloaded from my website www.TrishLaub.com.

🐞

Caregiver Agreements and Responsibilities
After a caregiver had been identified, interviewed and their background and references checked, we discussed the agreement and responsibilities necessary for becoming part of our care team. To be clear on our needs, my family created

a Caregiver Agreement that also identified the responsibilities of the job. It included:

- The client name
- The commencement date of the job
- The probationary period and terms
- The care location
- The care time (day/time) commitment
- Compensation and terms of receiving it such as completion of a timesheet
- Responsibilities required, but not limited to
- Agreements regarding completing specific tasks and terms for requesting scheduling changes
- Dress code
- Identification of any previously scheduled time off
- Agreement to amount of time off including holidays
- Terms of termination of services: amount of time of notification and terms for immediate termination
- Caregiver address and phone
- Caregiver signature with date
- Client signature and date

Daily Objectives and Requirements for Each Shift
We had four daily objectives:

Our parents are safe.
Our parents' meds are given correctly and on time.
Our parents are clean, fed and happy.
Our parents receive considerate and respectful care with every consideration for privacy.

Prior to stating the requirements for each shift, we stated that the caregivers collectively (including my sisters and me) were a team and as such needed to work together. For example, if one of us used an item it was to be cleaned if necessary and put back in the right place so that the next person could find it.

We also stated our strategy for contacting us, in order to prevent too much or too little communication and escalation of urgent communication. We encouraged all communication including questions, concerns, suggestions, compliments and complaints.

- Nonurgent communication: an email copied to my sisters and me
- Urgent communication regarding compromised health or safety or the need for an immediate answer: a call to me or my sisters. (We provided the order in which to call us). We promised a call or text within 5 minutes, after which the caregiver was to contact the next on the list.
- An emergency: call 9-1-1 and then call me or my sisters. They were to leave a voice message and then text "9-1-1" to each of us.

👀 👀 Because I knew that if a caregiver was calling me it was important, I changed the ringtone for all of our caregivers to an obnoxious blaring alarm that could not be missed.

Finally, we identified the requirements for each shift. These included required paperwork, the checking of medication supplies, care procedures, food preparation and storage, end-of-day preparation for the following day and shift completion.

The Caregiver Book

While caregiving is about providing care for another person, it requires entering another person's living space. In addition to all the responsibilities for care, learning the ins and outs of another person's living space can be overwhelming. The living space may be a single room in a facility that provides meal preparation and housekeeping, or it may be a large home consisting of many rooms involving meal preparation and light housekeeping. My family provided personal training for each caregiver as they entered our parents' home. We also chose to create a Caregiver Book that included the information and was placed in a central location for easy reference in the future. It included:

- <u>Welcome!</u>
  Welcome to the caregivers, into my parents' home and onto my parents' care team

- <u>Introduction to the clients</u>
  A brief history of my parents: who they are and what is important to them

- <u>Family</u>
  A list of immediate family members (including spouses and children) and their relationship to the client

- <u>In General</u>
  Important details in regard to each parent: Dad had a pacemaker, my parents wore hearing aids, they each had arthritis. Mom and Dad had food restrictions, Dad had food and medication allergies etc.

- <u>Shift Start and End</u>
  What was to happen at the start, during and end of each shift

- Pay Cards
  The process for filling out pay cards and receiving payment and any reimbursements
- Devices
  Any equipment or devices available to assist in caregiving, such as a motion sensor, audio monitor, call bell etc.
- Medication
  All notes regarding medications, administration and procedures
- Food
  Meal times and notes on food preparation and restrictions
- Hygiene
  Specific notes regarding the use of gloves during care, clothing preferences for each parent, bathing regimen and any other pertinent information
- Exercises
  Any exercise each parent was required or wanted to do and how to motivate them to do the work
- Typical Day
  Complete details of a typical day including the morning, afternoon, evening and bedtime activities and routines complete with examples of meals
- Household
  Specifics in regard to the household, such as shopping for and handling groceries, replenishment of supplies, using the air conditioner, and refuse and recycling
- Professionalism
  Our perspective on professionalism, always required toward the client and family but also essential toward team members

- <u>Alzheimer's Disease</u> (or any other disease that requires special consideration)
  Information about Alzheimer's, and our philosophy on it, because Dad had the disease
- <u>Some Final Notes</u>
  A reminder that it is difficult for a client to allow a caregiver into their home, and that respecting our parents' previous way of life was critical
- <u>Contact info</u>
  Client address, client name and contact info, immediate family member names and contact info and any next door neighbors names and contact info
- <u>Emergency/Medical/Medication Info</u>
  Procedure for contacting 9-1-1 (some senior living residences have procedures), preferred hospital (paramedics may determine to which hospital a patient will be taken depending on the emergency), information the medical providers need to know immediately, current medications, allergies to medication, power of attorney, advanced directive, insurance information and medical providers (PCP and specialists)

After a short time of use, my family and the caregiver team began to refer to the Caregiver Book as the "red book." We placed copies of each of my parents' driver's license, Medicare card, power of attorney and advanced directive documents in the back of the notebook. It ultimately became known as the Emergency Information Book. Anytime a parent went to a facility, the red book came with us, as it contained all of the information necessary for a facility admission.

Monthly Schedules

You may be the only caregiver or you may be one of a team. In any case it is helpful to provide a weekly schedule of care to the person requiring care. It helps them have a visual reminder of when someone will be available and present to assist them, and who that will be. As I've said, toward the end of my time providing care, I was scheduling nine caregivers in any given week. I chose to do the monthly schedules in a calendar format and make them available to my parents, sisters and the caregiving team. Any changes to that schedule were identified on the calendar that hung in the kitchen, using neon stickers to stand out as an exception. Below is a black and white example of our monthly schedule. Each caregiver had a unique bright color to represent their shift. The schedule helped everyone to literally stay on the same page.

~ May 2013 ~

Sunday	Monday	Tuesday	Wednesday	Thursday	Friday	Saturday
28 DEBBIE 9:00-	29 DEBBIE	30 DEBBIE	1 ANN 9-7, MW 7-9	2 MARGERY 9:00-	3 MARGERY	4 MARGERY
REGINA O.N. - 7 am	REGINA O.N. - 7 am	PATTI O.N - 10 am	BARB O.N.-7:30 am	SHERRY O.N. - 7	NANC O.N.-8 am	SHERRY O.N. - 7
7 am -10 am	7 am - 9 am	SHERRY 10 am - 2	7:30 am - 9 am	7 am - 10 am	ANN 8 am - 1 p.m.*	ANN 8 am - 12 am*
SHERRY 10 am - 3	PATTI 9 am - O.N.	2 pm - 5 pm	RUTH 9 am - 5 pm	SHERRY 10 am - 5	Ann 5 pm - 9 pm	Ann 4 pm - 7 pm *
3 pm - 7 pm		BARB 5 pm - O.N.	5 pm - 9 pm	NANC 5 pm - O.N.	SHERRY 9 pm -	REGINA 7 pm - O.N.
REGINA 7 pm -			SHERRY 9 pm -O.N.		(Kendrick 11:40	
	(Wendel 1:30 Patti)					
5 DEBBIE 9:00-	6 DEBBIE	7 DEBBIE	8 DEBBIE	9 MARGERY 9:00-	10 MARGERY	11 MARGERY
REGINA O.N. - 7 am	MARGERY O.N. - 8	SHERRY O.N. - 7	MARGERY O.N.- 8	BARB O.N. - 7:30	NANC O.N. - 8 am	SHERRY O.N. - 7
RUTH 8 am - 11 am	RUTH 8 am - 11 am	RUTH 8 am - 11 am	ANN 8 am - 11 am	ANN 8 am - 11 am	ANN 8 am - 11 am	ANN 8 am - 12 pm
5 pm - 8 pm	SHERRY 5 pm - 8	SHERRY 5 pm - 8	Ann 5 pm - 9 pm	NANC 5 pm - 9 pm	Ann 5 pm - 9 pm	Ann 4 pm - 7 pm
MARGERY 8 pm-	SHERRY 9 pm - O.N.	MARGERY 8 pm-	BARB 9 pm - O.N.	NANC 9 pm - O.N.	SHERRY 9 pm -	ANGEL 8 pm - O.N.
12 DEBBIE 9:00-	13 DEBBIE	14 DEBBIE	15 DEBBIE	16 MARGERY 9:00-	17 MARGERY	18 MARGERY
ANGEL O.N. - 9 am	MARGERY O.N. - 8	PATTI O.N. - 9 am	MARGERY O.N.- 8	BARB O.N. - 7:30	NANC O.N. - 8 am	BARB O.N. - 8:00
PATTI 9 am - 1 pm	RUTH 8 am - 12 pm	RUTH 9 am - 12 pm	ANN 8 am - 12 pm	ANN 8 am - 12 pm	ANN 8 am - 12 pm	ANN 8 am - 12 pm
NANC						
BARB 5 pm - 9 pm	PATTI 5 pm - 9 pm	RUTH 5 pm - 8 pm	Ann 4 pm - 7 pm	NANC 5 pm - 9 pm	Ann 4 pm - 7 pm	Ann 4 pm - 7 pm *
MARGERY 9 pm -	PATTI 9 pm - O.N.	MARGERY 8 pm-	BARB 7(?) pm - O.N.	NANC 9 pm - O.N.	BARB 7(?) pm -	ANGEL 8 pm - O.N.
	(Wendel 2:30 Patti)		(Evox Dad 1:30 Patti)			NANC 9 pm - O.N.

149

Daily Logs

Daily logs were likely *the most important tool we used to manage our parents' care.* When providing care, working with illness and disease, and administering medications, it is imperative that as few mistakes as possible are made. For example, one of my Dad's medications had to be administered within a small window of time to be effective. If it was administered even 10 minutes late, he would be miserable and most likely awake all night.

Also the accurate recording of bodily function allowed us to be pre-emptive in getting treatment for symptoms and illnesses, such as UTIs and colds, that would otherwise have been more significant due to my parents' ages.

Below is an examples of our daily logs. Most of it applies to any patient, some of it was patient specific. We put the pages in a three-ring notebook. Placing the first page you see on the left and second page on the right. That way we could look at all of the information for the day at once. Again, these pages were color coded to help identify what was most important.

See pages 152 and 153.

Shift-Turnover Sheets

With nine caregivers on the schedule in a week, there was a lot of coming and going. When one parent or the other was in crisis, had a new diagnosis or needed special care, things could change quickly. It was critical that the next caregiver could get up to speed fast. Prior to the end of a caregiver shift, they were required to fill out the Shift-Turnover Sheet. The next caregiver arrived 15 minutes before their shift started to review the shift-turnover sheet with the caregiver preparing to leave. **Every** caregiver, *including my sisters and me*, filled out the shift-turnover sheets and reviewed them with the caregiver arriving for the next shift.

SHIFT TURNOVER SHEET
If there are any concerns about anything that may have happened on a shift other than your own or to schedule time off, please contact Jean or someone in the Moore family.
TURNOVER NOTES BY: Caregiver: Shift Dates:
TURNOVER NOTES GIVEN TO: Caregiver:
Events/Episodes
Work in Progess (laundry)
Food (leftovers, pods) *** please remember to label and date all food
Newly Scheduled/Reminder Events
Concerns

Left-hand page of Daily Log

Client Name:		
*** ALL changes to meds must be highlighed/circled. This INCLUDES TYLENOL and PRN!		

SPECIAL PROCEDURE	Time	Inits

MEDICATIONS	6:00 AM	

BREAKFAST	10:00 AM	

AFTERNOON	2:00 PM	

DINNER	6:00 PM	

BEDTIME	10:00 PM	

MEDICATIONS	2:00 AM	

DAY/DATE:		CAREGIVER:		

AM/PM CARE:	Time	Inits	Self	Assist
Time up				
AM CARE				
Bath				
Body Lotion				
Traumeel				
Brush Teeth				
Comb Hair				
Dressing				
Temp and BP				
"normal" is:				

BREAKFAST MEDS		

MIDDAY			
BP (if am unusual)			

EXERCISE	YES / NO

NAP	YES / NO

SEE NOTES	YES / NO

DINNER Meds		

PM CARE			
Prepartion for Bed			
Time to bed			

BEDTIME Meds		

END OF DAY:		
Complete Daily Logs		
Fill out Timesheet		

TASKS:		
P/U newspaper, aft 8 am		
Meal serve/clear		
Beds/Sheets (both)		
Laundry		
P/U mail/pkgs		
Shredding		
Take recycling out		

Right-hand page of Daily Log

CLIENT NAME:					SUMMARY (DATE) _____		
MEALS:						% Eaten	# Drinks
Breakfast:							
Lunch:							
Snack:							
Dinner:							
Notes:						TOTAL=	

MOBILITY:	Please note, ALWAYS ATTEMPT USING THE WALKER before using the transfer chair!					
Walker:		#of time	Notes:			
Wheelchair:		#of times				
MOOD:	Normal	Notes:				
	YES / NO					
ENERGY:	Normal	Notes:				
	YES / NO					
NOTES:	Time	use YELLOW highlighter on URINE VOID times, ORANGE highlighter on SOLID VOID				

Caregiver Team Newsletters

As our care team grew it became more and more difficult to effectively disseminate important information. Out of this came the caregiver team newsletters.

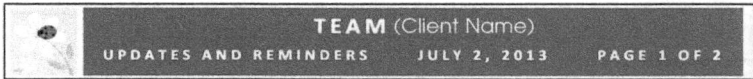

TEAM (Client Name)

UPDATES AND REMINDERS   JULY 2, 2013   PAGE 1 OF 2

Each newsletter had a color banner on the top with "TEAM" followed by my parents' last name. Underneath that we stated "Updates and Reminders", the date, and page of page, eg.) Page 1 of 2.

The newsletters varied in content but included:
- Reminders, such as providing more detail on the daily log sheets
- Fun quizzes on aspects of their jobs such as, "What are the objectives of your job?" "What times are the client's meds given?" and "What is the client's favorite food?"
- Updates on procedures
- Updates on caregiver team members, including new hires and those with whom we had terminated services We expressed that we wished all previous caregivers well, regardless of who terminated service. We supported caregiver relationships outside of work, as future jobs are often acquired through networking, but reminded everyone that all information about their job with my parents was to remain private.
- Acknowledgment of caregiver birthdays and special events such as weddings and births
- Differentiation between reminders and new information

- Notes specific to a shift: 24-hour vs 12-hour and day vs night
- Addressed any job functions that needed improvement in a way that was not pointed at any one caregiver. Reminders were always addressed to the entire team.

Our newsletter always closed with a compliment about the caregivers' skill and services and an expression of gratitude for them.

When we had a new newsletter, it was placed in the front of each caregiver's folder. If the information was critical, we included a page that required a signature indicating that the caregiver had read the newsletter. That page was required to be signed and returned to us by the end of their shift.

The feedback we received from our caregiver team was that they truly appreciated our newsletter. Some felt that it created a more cohesive team. Others felt that the newsletters were not only informational but also educational.

Considerations at a Housing Complex

My parents lived in a condo in a complex. It was run by a homeowners' association board and managed by a property management company. I mention all of this because it ultimately required us to follow certain procedures that we hadn't previously known.

- An access code was required to enter the parking lot in order to prevent public parking. Initially we requested that the caregivers call our unit when they arrived for a shift, requiring us to buzz them into the complex. This avoided having to give each caregiver our personal access code. After the frequent failure of the buzzer and the many times the working caregiver was assisting a parent and unable to respond to the buzzer, we were able to request and **obtain a caregiver access code** in addition to our personal access code. Each caregiver now had the ability to enter the parking lot without being dependent on someone in our unit buzzing them in. This was particularly nice when shift changes were early in the morning.

- Although parking was available for our guests, we were eventually required to identify our caregivers when they were parked while working. As a caregiver could park and leave their car for three or four 24-hour periods, it sometimes became necessary to contact the caregiver to move their car in the event of snow plowing. To facilitate this process, **the property management company made placards for the caregiver vehicles** stating how the caregiver could be reached if necessary, and we provided each caregiver's license plate number. The caregivers were then required to place the placard in the front window of their vehicle every time they arrived to work.

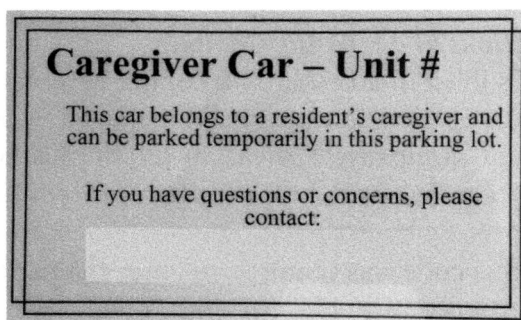

Caregiver Car – Unit

This car belongs to a resident's caregiver and can be parked temporarily in this parking lot.

If you have questions or concerns, please contact:

- There was **a procedure for calling 9-1-1 and the property management company wanted to be notified.** Emergency vehicles had access to the parking lot system but we always sent someone out to wait for the vehicle and to direct the paramedics to our unit.

- **The property management company also required being notified if the unit was going to be empty** more than a couple of days. This allowed the property manager to keep an eye on the unit.

- Living in a condo complex is community living. **It is important for family member and caregivers to be respectful of the community** by being respectful of the property, courteous to the residents and compliant with the HOA and property-management rules. This includes something as simple as properly preparing the garbage before it goes down the garbage shoot.

Setting up Shop at Home
Being organized and having supplies easily accessible was not only important to ensuring quality care but also very helpful. We evaluated where everything necessary for care would be best located for purposes of consolidation and ease of access, to allow for as much of the home to remain unaffected as possible.

Below are some of the things that were helpful to my family.
- Kitchen
  Because of the way my parents' home was designed, the kitchen was a central area of activity. That is where we kept the Emergency Information Book (which also housed the Caregiver Book), the daily logs, shift-turnover sheets and medications, all of which could be used while overseeing the preparation of a meal. A copy of the monthly caregiver schedule hung next to the

regular wall calendar on which we placed neon stickers identifying the name of all substitute caregivers to make all changes to the printed monthly schedule visible to everyone.

We used the front of the refrigerator for quick access to important information such as emergency phone numbers and procedures and medical provider information, and attached a white board on which we could write the status of a replenishment request.

We placed a list of frozen foods available for preparation on the side of the refrigerator, along with a pad of paper on which to write items for the next grocery shop.

Because Mom and Dad had food restrictions, we identified foods that they could not eat. A bag of clementines was marked indicating that they could not be given to Mom. Any product containing aspartame was marked so that it would not be given to Dad.

Because we had so many people in and out of the kitchen, it was especially important to keep it clean. The refrigerator had to be cleaned often. That meant not only throwing out any food that had expired, but also cleaning the physical refrigerator which had sustained drips and spills during the week. The stovetop and microwave were to be cleaned after each use and the floor was to be cleaned anytime there was a spill, or at least daily.

- Medications
  We purchased a medium plastic storage box with a drawer in it. We divided the inside of the box in half crosswise with a piece of cardboard. All current

medications were stored in the front of the box. All refills were stored in the back of the box. When we received refills, we placed orange stickers on the original bottle and on the refills. If there were three bottles of the same medication, we placed a "#1 of 3" on the original bottle, and a "#2 of 3" and "3 of 3" on the two new refill bottles. When the current bottle was empty, we took the refill bottle next in numerical order, changed its number to "#1 of 2", and adjusted what had been the third bottle to reflect being the second bottle. That helped us to keep track of our inventory and to be aware of when we needed a refill, leaving enough time to get a new prescription if necessary. We allowed 15 days for filling a new prescription.

Initially, we were able to preload weekly medication boxes and administer the medications at the designated time. As care became more complex, we chose to prepare the medication for each administration time immediately prior to that time. This helped us ensure that we accurately dispensed the most current medications and up-to-date dosages.

As far as preparing medications for administration, we had a protocol which everyone followed.
1. Using the daily log sheet, find each medication and remove it from the medication box. Line the medication up in the same order as they appear on the daily log sheet.
2. Working in the order of the bottles, check the patient name, medication name and dosage on each bottle to the daily log sheet.
3. Opening one bottle at a time, remove the medication and place it in a dish. When you are done with that bottle, close the bottle and turn it upside down.

4. Continue with each bottle, turning each bottle over when you have removed the correct dosage.

5. When you have done this with every bottle, count the bottles and the medication in the dish. Verify that you have the correct number of pills. If not, find the error and correct it.

6. Finally, initial that you have prepared the medication.

7. When the medication is administered, write the time.

8. If for any reason the medication is administered by someone other than the person who prepared it, the person who administered the medication must initial the daily log sheet too.

Our method of medication management worked for us, but today there are many alternatives. Large medication boxes with sections for holding morning, afternoon, evening and bedtime medications, for each day of the week or month, are available. These work if the person can load their own medications or if they have someone they trust to do it for them. Pillpack.com offers a pharmacy service which will provide your medications prepackaged by date and time of day.

👀👀 As I said in Chapter 8, whether or not a certified CNA can legally administer any or all medications is determined by state and whether the CNA has additional required training. Additional training and certification through a qualified medication-administration curriculum (QMAP) may be necessary. QMAP certification verification can be found by Googling "QMAP verification".

- Laundry Room
We created a Caregiver Communication Center (CCC) in the laundry room. Each caregiver was given a folder in which to keep important papers and past communications, and in which new communications were placed in the front. Critical communications required that the caregiver sign and return a sheet of acknowledgment that they read the communication, which was attached to the new document. Upon occasion, we also left little treats in their folders. In the CCC, we made available sheets on which they could write their comments, suggestions, tips and techniques. On top of the CCC was a box containing paycards on which they recorded their shift hours.,

👀👀 Paycards also allowed for recording any reimbursable personal expenses, such as mileage when they used their personal car for work-related errands or appointments or the expense of an item purchased for our household.

We added shelves in the laundry room to create a place to store extra supplies such as paper goods, garbage bags and care products. We stocked extra of all supplies so that a caregiver never ran out of a supply in the middle of the night.

The laundry room was available for our caregivers to do our parents' laundry in case of an accident, or for our 24-hour caregivers to do their own laundry.

- Bedroom
The master bedroom had been the place where both of my parents had slept for many years. It was already set

up to their liking and for comfort. When we had to create a second bedroom for my Mom, in what had been the dining room, we went to great lengths to make it feel cozy and organized. We purchased nice pretty sheets, used a lightweight flannel blanket and placed a Styrofoam roller under the sheets at the bottom of the bed. There were other devices, such as a hospital bed, and supplies that we used that were immensely helpful. (See Chapter 11.) Mom had to use a commode at that point and it was stored away from the bed when not in use and always kept clean. We placed one of our large family photos, one which we took to each facility, where it was visible to Mom and our caregivers. We used shelves and plastic storage bins to keep her medically necessary supplies organized, out of sight and easily accessible to caregivers.

We put significant thought into my mom's move to another room, to prevent contamination of Dad via a shared bedroom or bathroom. While Mom wasn't happy about it, the dining room offered privacy, already having a door between it and the kitchen. Its proximity to the kitchen made it convenient when Mom needed food or fluids while in bed, and it was an easy source of water. We purchased inexpensive but beautiful privacy screens to stretch across the opening between the dining room and the living room, as Mom did not want a visitor to know that she was sleeping in the dining room.

- Caregiver bedroom
  We made every effort to make our caregivers feel comfortable, especially those who did 24-hour shifts and slept there. We provided each overnight caregiver with their own pretty sheets and towels, as well as a large

storage bin in which to store them and other personal items between shifts and a bathroom bucket to store their toothbrush and soap. We provided a TV and Internet service and power strips in the room. And we considered it their private room, which we did not enter unless necessary and only with their permission.

Things That We Found Helpful

Some days are just bad days, that's all.
You have to experience sadness
to know happiness,
and I remind myself that not every day
is going to be a good day,
that's just the way it is!
Dita Von Teese

Caregiving is a tough job. It is not for the weak. Even when I prepared and did everything according to plan, some days just didn't go well. I learned a lot through trial and error, and in the beginning, error was the majority of my experience. But, every day I got up and was determined to do my best. Sometimes my best was not great, but it was the best that I could do on that day.

Courage does not always roar.
Sometimes courage is the quiet voice
at the end of the day saying,
"I will try again tomorrow."
Unknown

There were literally hundreds of tips and techniques we amassed as we cared for our parents. Below are just a few that have not already been mentioned and that were particularly important.

👀 See Chapter 12 for tips on how we handled specific medical issues.

- Be sure to *have seniors sign documents* while they can. If legal documents need to be changed, do not wait.
- When we were in a restaurant, we asked that they bring water or other *drinks in small, lightweight glasses.*
- Due to hearing loss, we found that my dad could hear us better if *we spoke in a lower tone of voice* and faced him directly, so that he could see our face when we spoke.
- Laying on a hearing aid is miserable. *We always removed our parents' hearing aids from the ear on which they were going to lie.* The trick was to remember to put it back in afterward.
- My dad perceived that we were driving faster than we were and it made him nervous. *We had to be more aware of our driving* so that he would be comfortable.
- When my mom's blood pressure was taken digitally, it would be inaccurate. Many seniors find that unless their *blood pressure is taken manually,* the result will be falsely elevated.
- When we purchased cards for our dad, who had Alzheimer's, we looked for *cards with large print and few words.* We also continued to purchase cards and gifts for Dad to give Mom.
- We *always re-evaluated our situation,* all diagnoses and every procedure.
- My parents got *angry if they were rushed or treated roughly.* Treat others as you want to be treated. Along that line, we spoke directly to our parents, and never spoke about them as though they were not present.

- In a facility where a person is wearing a hospital gown that is open in the back, *place a second gown on them in the opposite direction* before they walk anywhere.
- When ill, my parents' ability to comprehend information or direction was compromised. The uses of *three-word sentences* was immensely effective.
- We learned that each day of immobility, such as in bed, required an average of *three days of recovery* often requiring physical and occupational therapy.
- Having family members who were local *drop in unannounced* kept everyone on their toes.
- We received *training from PTs and OTs* on how to properly move our parents, including how to assist someone in going to the floor in the event that they can no longer stand.
- Moving or transferring people takes time. Be patient and move slowly.
  - 🐞🐞🐞 When raising someone up from a lying position in bed, many people grab the person's arms and pull them up. Please do not. Instead, slide your arm behind their upper back (not their shoulders or neck) similar to giving them a one-arm hug. You may have to put your knee up on the bed to do this so you don't strain your own back! Ask them to tuck their chin and roll toward you. This method allows the weight of their body to assist in raising their chest and puts no pressure on their joints. My experience was that while in the hospital, the staff often used to raise Mom or Dad by their neck (really dangerous) and/or shoulders (painful), which not only hurt them but also made them understandably angry.
  - 🐞🐞🐞 If you must move the lower body of someone with knee issues, wrap your arm underneath their thighs, never their knees. This

keeps the pressure off of their knees and allows you to move their lower body as one unit. Also, using the bed pad to gently roll someone onto a hip (so that they are fully on their side, hips stacked) helps their hips and back because they are not twisted into a position that is half on their back and half on their side.

o 👀 👀 👀 When lifting someone, *lift with your hand not fingers*. Otherwise the fingers become like painful claws that dig into the person.

- When doing any procedure, *assume it will take longer than you anticipate*. Take your time. As bodies get older, they are more delicate and procedures are more painful.

- Dad was a large man and therefore we instructed our family members and caregivers not to lift him. When Dad slipped and fell at night, we were able to call the non-emergency phone number for the police department and request a *lift assist*. Many fire departments provide the service for seniors free of charge. Be aware that the paramedics will do a quick assessment for injures, and often recommend that the person who has fallen be taken to the ED. The family can decline that service.

- My sisters and I were *collective medical power of attorneys*. Whichever one of us was present when a decision had to be made, provided that our parents were unable to make their own decision, had the authority to make the decision. Whenever possible, the sister who was present contacted the other two sisters for concurrence on a decision. *Collective decision making* not only provided assurance that it was the best possible decision but also reduced the stress of being solely responsible for the decision.

- Whenever getting in or out of the car, my parents would grab the car door, which would then start to close on them. Always *put pressure against the car door, pushing it away from the car*, as soon as someone attempts getting in or out of the car.
- Sometimes we needed an ambulance to transport Mom on a stretcher. Other times we used an ambulance thinking it was the only way to transport Mom in a wheelchair when she could not transfer in and out of it to ride in a car. We learned that there are *wheelchair taxis and vans,* which are much less expensive than an ambulance. Google: your town followed by "wheelchair taxi."
- *Google everything*, every business name with which you might work and every person's name involved in care. A facility arranged for my dad to be transported to a medical appointment via an ambulance. The ambulance attendants were very unprofessional, disrespectful to my dad and in fact caused him pain. I googled the company to find horrific reviews of the company. We notified the facility that we would refuse to use the company in the future.
- Eye drops are more easily administered if you slightly pull down on the lower lid, creating a pocket for the drop to fall into.
- Some medications are available for sublingual use, under the tongue or inside the cheek. It was helpful when my parents couldn't sit up to take a pill.
- As I mentioned before, we tied non-skid socks to the end of a hospital bed so that we could always find them.
- Plastic spoons taped to each headrail closest to the part nearest the center of the bed helped to keep oxygen tubing from getting caught on things.

- We used a chip clip to hold the back of a shirt or nightgown up out of the toilet.
- We brought flowers, balloons and sometimes treats to our parents especially when they were in a medical facility. We were caregivers, but *we were daughters first.*
- We purchased *grocery store gift cards* that could be used by our caregivers when doing grocery shopping for my parents' household. Caregivers were to provide us with a receipt showing use of the card, and to notify us when there was $50 left on the card so that we could replenish it.

  🐞 🐞 Many grocery stores offer pick-up and/or delivery service for orders that are either called into the store or placed online.
- We collected and *washed all the hand towels* at the end of each day.
- We *continually looked for helpful items,* such as large print check registers, and more effective supplies.
- We always remembered that *slowly and gently massaging the head or back* is very soothing.

🐞 🐞 🐞 *A Most Meaningful Life* presents a specific strategy and additional tips for assisting someone with dementia or memory loss.

Dignified Care
Dignified care goes way beyond the basic rights of a person: to be housed, fed, clothed, and not abused. It goes beyond dignified medical care. It speaks to the basics decencies of human interaction such as being treated kindly and with respect, and to the need for every person to feel cared for and valuable.

> Kind words can be short and easy to speak
> but their echoes are truly endless.
> Mother Teresa

While we followed Mom and Dad's medical treatment plans, we also observed and made additions to their daily regimen based on our observations, conferring with medical providers first when necessary. We found that the following were helpful to my parents.

- Probiotics, to promote immune health and to deter the negative effects of antibiotics
- Vitamin D, as my parents were no longer outdoors as much as previously, their vitamin D levels decreased. This can be seen when the person is less energetic and can result in depression. We had their vitamin D levels checked and then supplemented it.
- D-Mannose was given proactively to prevent UTIs.
- Coconut oil was instrumental in improving Dad's cognitive function. Dad had Alzheimer's.
- Antidepressant - often with serious illness, especially dementia, it becomes necessary to treat depression
- Complementary treatments - Evox (an emotional reframing technique) was immensely helpful for my Dad when he got stuck in an emotional loop caused by Alzheimer's. There are other techniques such as EMDR, acupuncture and body work that are helpful.

Things that were part of their daily lives before they were required care were continued even when they were bedridden. We continued:

- Brushing their teeth
- Keeping their hair clean, brushing and styling it

- Wearing nice night clothes including a robe and slippers if desired
- Always wearing **clean** clothes, anything that got dirty was promptly changed. They also wore what they always had. Dad always wore a button-down shirt and khaki pants, and never a t-shirts or jeans.
- Offering a warm cloth for hands and face make them instantly feel better
- Doing anything that made them feel important

I recently saw an "ad," a video, by Gillette for their new assisted-shaving razor. I love everything about the video: the respect in "good morning sir;" the love between parent and child; the son's perspective on caring and reassurance for his father; and the care and patience with which he groomed his father each day. It reminded me of when my husband and brothers-in-law would shave my Dad. He would sit in his recliner and let them carefully and gently run an electric razor all over his face. Dad sat there looking like he was getting the best straight razor shave of his life and it made him relaxed and peaceful. It was a gift that the men in my family could offer my dad that made Dad feel like a pampered king. It was a ritual that continued even when Dad was bedridden. View the video: https://youtu.be/WjjhcdcBkK4 and visit www.GilletteTreo.com.

We were able to find in-home, or mobile, services that were invaluable.
- A senior care specialist who made house visits
- A nail/foot RN, necessary for nail and foot care
- A dental hygienist who did teeth cleaning while Mom was in bed

- A hair stylist who would cut and style Mom's hair after we washed her hair while she was in bed
- A nail technician who did manicures and pedicures
- A massage therapist

To find services, Google "in home," "mobile" or "service for seniors" followed by the service you want.

Although we did not use this service, there is a non-profit organization of high school and college girls who provide complimentary companionship, manicures and makeovers to women living in senior homes. They have 100 chapters around the country. Google: Glamour Gals.

> No act of kindness,
> no matter how small,
> is ever wasted.
> Aesop

Finally, we treated Mom and Dad as we always had – with dignity. We always put their welfare first, were polite and respectful. We listened to music, watched TV shows and movies, and talked about things they liked. It never mattered to me what I was doing with them, it was about being with them. If my sisters or I saw something we thought they would like while we were out, we brought it home for them as a special little treat that let them know that we were thinking about them even when we were away. We found ways to tell them how important they were to us, how appreciative we were for all that they had done for each us during our lives, and how much we loved them and always would.

The Importance of Music

One of the only activities that activates, stimulates and uses the entire brain is music. I found that magical things happened whenever I put music familiar to my parents on in their home. Regardless of the time of day, my mom relaxed as she had so many times when she put "her music" on at 5:00 p.m. every evening. In spite of having Alzheimer's, Dad instantly knew every word to every song and each instrument played. The music brought each parent back to some memory of where they were when they heard the song. Music was an invaluable tool to anchoring my parents to the day and to us, as well as bringing them joy.

In a Sept. 9, 2013 post on his blog, *Searching for the Mind* Jon Lieff MD states, "Music not only uniquely uses all of the brain, but stimulates neuroplasticity changes, which increase learning of all types. The brain is uniquely responsive to sound, taking extremely complex multiple qualities of timbre, rhythm and melody and making them one sound that we hear, stimulating memories, emotions and learning. The unique qualities of music in human life are just now being appreciated in science."

During the days that each parent was unconscious and transitioning to the end of their life, we played music: Mom's favorite song and instrumental music that soothed Dad. I will forever remember that music.

A Word About Stress

I only touched on stress in Chapter 1. It is well documented that long-term stress can lead to serious health problems, ranging from depression and anxiety to heart and chronic disease. For my sisters and me, it was a real concern. We spent 2 ½ years managing and providing care for both of our parents. I did the best that I could to care for myself but honestly, there were many times I put my parents' welfare far before my own. I got way too little sleep and ate what I could on the run, which was often not very healthy. In July of 2013, my sisters and I held a care-team meeting during which we discussed many topics regarding the care of our parents, as well as our concerns about our long-term health.

The very next morning I came across a video that supported what I had felt all along. It was a Ted Talk given by Kelly McGonigal called "How to make stress your friend." (www. Ted.com/talks, search "Kelly McGonigal".) She spoke about the effect of caregiving on the caregiver's health. The bottom line was that caregivers who willingly made the choice to provide care suffered far less negative effects than those who felt obligated to provide care. She said that in fact, caring creates resilience and stress is affected by how we think and act. It made sense to me, as professional caregivers are able to provide care without suffering compromised health and it is, after all, the professional caregiver's choice to provide care. The vido said that it all comes down to perspective, whether you are willingly providing care and moving with the flow of care, or you are providing care begrudgingly and fighting the process.

Working hard for something we don't care about
is called stress.
Working hard for something we love
is called passion.
Simon Sinek

Although I was completely willing to provide care, at the end of 2 ½ years I was completely depleted: physically, mentally, emotionally and spiritually. I had given everything to ensure that the two people who mattered most, the parents who had cared for me every time I needed care, were delivered the best possible care and the end-of-life that they desired. I did not suffer long-term illness, but it took me a year to even start to get back to my original baseline of health. It was a year that required patience, and complete acceptance of my need for self-care, in order to renourish my body, to refresh my mind, to process my emotions and to again allow my spirit to find a new path no longer based on caregiving.

When the Caregiving Job is Over
We hired 17 caregivers in 18 months. The majority were great. Those who chose to end their services, for a variety of reasons, were wished well on their way knowing that we provided a letter of recommendation and were always available to be a reference. Those who were not a fit for us were terminated immediately, and still wished well on their search for the right fit. Those who were with us at each parent's end of life, and literally overnight found themselves without work, were compensated with additional pay. These caregivers had provided care for a period of time and had bonded with my parents and my family. They deserved paid time to grieve, as well as time to find another client.

Many of our caregivers became like family. They lived the final years of my parents' lives with us. They saw the good and bad, the happy and sad, shared their birthdays and holidays with us and returned for their next shift to continue to provide dignified care for my parents. In the years since we have worked together, I have helped many of our former caregivers find work with good clients. I have taken reference calls and written additional letters. Some are in touch at holidays and birthdays, and others share their current news. Some I have had the good fortune to occasionally meet for coffee or lunch, some I have been able to be supportive of in their personal lives and with one I have shared the process of writing.

Caregivers are the unsung heroes of those in need of care.

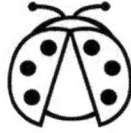

We spend billions of dollars
on trying to prevent aging,
but aging is a process
that begins at birth.
Trish Laub

Chapter 10

SENIOR CARE ...

considerations as we age

Generally, by the time you are Real,
most of your hair has been loved off,
and your eyes drop out
and you get loose in the joints
and very shabby.
But these things don't matter at all,
because once you are Real
you can't be ugly,
except to people who don't understand.
The Velveteen Rabbit, Margery Williams Bianco

My former father-in-law used to say that aging was not for wussies. He was a man who enlisted in WWII at the age of 17 and survived Omaha Beach, not only served President Eisenhower but shared a drink with him, saw Roosevelt's funeral, attended Truman's birthday party, and shook the hand of President Kennedy. He started as a self-trained carpenter and would buy a piece of property, build the house literally above him as he lived in the basement, and sell it and repeat the process again. He went on to be a self-made construction contractor, having worked his way up from his start as a carpenter, and ended up building much of a town in Ohio. He knew challenge and difficulty, and rose above it all to say that of all things, age was a bugger.

The classification as a senior can vary, identified for some purposes as 50+, others 60, and still others 62 or 65. The term senior is not synonymous with "old." Old is a state of mind.

I have known 20-somethings who I have thought were old, and people like my parents, who were in their 90s but never old. Their bodies may have gotten old, but they had not.

"OLD" is when you give up.
Until then,
you are spectacular.
Unknown

We age, and our body and brain eventually wear out and are no longer useful. Although Dad was not old, he used to ask me, "Why am I in this cumbersome body?" While heartbreaking, I understood his frustration.

I have said before, in regard to Alzheimer's, that people are not their disease. Nor are people disposable just because their body or brain have grown old and are less functional.

If you listen around the dementia,
past the weakened bodies and into their hearts,
you'll hear their stories.
Marky Olson, *Caregiving for Your Elderly Parents*

Senior care requires different considerations than care for others.

Medical Care
Medical Providers and Services
As the senior population grows in the United States, there are more medical providers who specialize in the care of seniors, a specialty called geriatric medicine. This specialty allows them to better interact with seniors. In some cases,

medical practices that specialize in senior care will even send a medical provider to the home of the senior.

> I hope that all medical providers are able
> to feel a connection that we cannot see,
> and that each has known a patient
> that they truly loved.
> I hope that they always know
> that their abilities and actions
> can change a patient's life.
> Trish Laub

As the medical care of a senior becomes more complex, and the senior becomes more vulnerable and sometimes even frail, it is especially important that a medical provider does the following:

1. Always introduces themself
2. Sees the person as an individual and respects that the family knows the patient's medical history
3. Addresses the patient and looks directly at them on their eye level
4. Strives to know the patient
5. Knows their audience and how to speak with the patient and the family
6. Listens with the intention to learn, not respond
7. Diagnoses the medical condition

Because of the complexities of illness that many seniors experience, it is important to be familiar with two valuable services: palliative care and hospice care. In addition to being valuable, they are also two of the most misunderstood services. An extremely short explanation is that palliative care provides comfort for symptoms of serious illness and hospice care provides comfort to those no longer undergoing life-extending treatment. The topics of both palliative and hospice care, as well as end of life, are covered in detail in *Peaceful Endings*.

More medical services are available to seniors as well, including in-home urgent care; GoodRx.com, which is a resource for comparing prescription prices from different vendors; and Pillpack.com, which offers pharmacy services including pre-packing medications according to dosages. And, there are many apps that assist seniors with everything from medical advice to services and interpersonal communication.

Understanding Medications

Medications can save lives, that is true. But many are cost-prohibitive for seniors; others have side effects that sometimes create new problems. Many factors must be considered in deciding whether the benefits of a specific medication outweigh the negatives. Also working against us is the announcement of health breakthroughs and promotion of medications to consumers via media. It seems that every day there is a new recommendation and a retraction of a former one. It can leave us wondering who really knows what for sure, and what we are supposed to believe and do.

Honest Medicine, shattering the myths about aging and health care, by Donald J. Murphy, M.D. is an eye-opening book. It is a statement about the need to arm ourselves with information in order to tailor a medical plan that enables us to grow old healthfully. In his book, the first step is to understand the meaningful numbers behind the statistics that are presented to the consumer.

Before we get into the numbers used to represent medications, consider the confusion caused by the presentation of numbers without explanation. Let's take the example of milk. There is whole milk, 2%, 1%, and skim. I had never researched what it meant, but I based my milk choices on my perceived understanding of what the numbers meant. I thought that 2% meant that there was either 2% as opposed to a much larger percentage of fat in the milk or that it had 2 % less fat in it than whole milk. I assumed that about 1% milk as well. Both of my uninformed assumptions are wrong, and in fact the truth is a bit shocking to me.

MILK

PER Cup	Cup	Whole: 3.25%	2%	1%	skim
grams	245	8.2	5.2	2.6	0.4
percentage of fat		3.35%	2.12%	1.06%	0.16%
teaspoons of fat		1.5	1	0.5	0
calories from fat		45	30	15	0
less fat than whole milk			33%	66%	100%
less calories than whole milk			15	30	45
total calories		146	122	105	91

The percentage for each type of milk is based on the percentage of the weight of the milk that comes from fat. A 1-cup serving of whole milk is 245 grams, of which 8.2 grams are fat, meaning that 3.35 % of the milk's weight comes from fat. The fat accounts for 45 of the 146 calories in the cup of milk. There are 1.5 teaspoons of fat in a cup of whole milk.

Part of the confusion comes from calling whole milk whole instead of 3.35%. More of the misunderstanding is seen when you realize that 1% milk is ½ of the fat and ½ the calories from fat, but not ½ the total calories of 2% milk. It all makes sense when you understand on what the numbers are based and what they actually mean. In re-evaluating the numbers, I may decide that the difference between drinking 1% and 2% milk is not significant enough for me to care.

If understanding the numbers is this complicated in regard to milk, you can imagine that it is more so in regard to medical studies and statistics. Dr. Murphy explains that understanding medication effectiveness in relation to you, requires that you understand the following.

1. <u>Statistical significance</u> is based on a formula and indicates that a medical finding is real and not by chance. Keep in mind that the threshold of significance was arbitrarily chosen in the 1930s.

    For example, let's say there are two test groups of 1,000 participants, one given a medication to prevent heart attacks and one given a placebo. After a period of time the medication group shows that 10 people had heart attacks; the placebo group shows that 20 people had heart attacks. The difference in 10 people (1% of 1,000) and 20 people (2% of 1,000 people) is deemed significant. This is a statement that if the study were repeated with different groups of people, the results would be similar in 95% of the studies.

    Once deemed statistically significant, the results are often presented as *relative risk reduction*. In the study, the results showed 10 vs 20 people having heart attacks, or a 50% reduction. It would appear that if you took the medication, your chances of having a heart attack would be reduced by 50%. This is misleading. It is important to understand the clinical significance and resultant <u>individual risk-reduction</u> results.

2. <u>Clinical significance</u> relates to the *individual risk reduction,* or how much something reduces your chance for a bad outcome.

In the placebo group, 20 people had heart attacks and 980 did not. The medication group had 10 heart attacks, meaning that the medication would have helped only 10 of the 20 in the placebo group that had heart attacks. The absolute risk reduction is 1% (10 of 1,000), not 50%.

In short, Dr. Murphy says, "Statistically significant medical findings may or may not be clinically significant for you." The point is that it's important to speak with your medical provider and to truly understand the individual risk-reduction benefit of any medication. Only then can you compare the potential benefit with the cost and side effects, allowing you to determine whether it is a desirable addition to your medical plan.

Effects of Medications and Illnesses
I have learned through the care of my parents that bacteria and infections affect us differently as we age. A case in point is the symptoms of urinary tract infections (UTIs.) While Chapter 12 highlights several medical issues that are most prevalent in the senior population, there are additional issues, such as dehydration. Seniors often drink less water and more coffee (a diuretic) and, it is common for them to dehydrate when feeling poorly. The symptoms of dehydration can run from UTIs to compromised heart rate, and can be very painful and serious. While younger people do experience dehydration, they typically have a greater reserve from which to recover.

Medications can affect us differently as we age. The normal dosage of anti-diarrhea medications such as Lomotil and Imodium are known to cause confusion in seniors, while they do not in younger people. These medications prompt the questions whether it is healthy to take them to stop diarrhea without knowing the cause of it. Diarrhea is often the body's way of expelling that which it does not want. Sadly, these medications are available over the counter, allowing seniors easy access in an attempt to avoid the inconvenience and expense of seeking professional help. Perhaps over-the-counter anti-diarrhea medications are better used as a temporary measure, such as getting to the doctor without an accident, in order to be properly diagnosed and treated. Anti-diarrhea medications are not the only medications that affect seniors differently. Medications are metabolized more slowly as we age and can cause different results.

👀 👀 A medical provider stated to me that she prescribes ½ the normal dosage of anti-diarrhea medication for seniors. Check with your medical provider for their prescribed dosage of all medications.

Blood thinners may pose a bleeding risk for seniors. There are two types of blood thinners: those that lessen the process called coagulation by which the blood clots, and those that prevent blood-cell fragments from sticking to the walls of your blood vessels and each other. If a person on anti-coagulant blood thinners were to be seriously injured with resultant significant bleeding, it might not be possible to stop the bleeding without the use of an anticoagulant-reversal medication or treatment.

And, we all have seen the medication advertisements on TV, listing all the horrible side effects. Yet we believe that the side effects will never happen to us. The problem is that if certain side effects occur, the situation is serious. My family had an experience with Xarelto. Mom was sent home from an STACH on a blood thinner, because she had been immobile for several days. A few days after she returned home, I began to receive texts and calls from caregivers that there was blood mysteriously coming from Mom's colostomy stoma. After looking back at our notebooks, I realized that the onset of the symptom coincided with the start of Xarelto, which we immediately stopped after consulting with the doctor.

This section is merely provided to bring awareness to possible issues for the senior population.

👀 👀 I have discussed in other chapters the importance of not giving up control when a senior is in the ICU. (See Chapter 12, *Clostridium Difficile: C. diff.*) The family is the holder of the patient's history and medical details.

Medical Advice
Because of liability, medical providers sometimes do not answer the question "What do you think I should do?" We found that if we phrased the questions as, "If it were your parent, what would you do?" we would get an answer.

Medical Testing
Keep it in perspective. Just because a test is available, does not mean that you should do it. Medical testing can provide information that is helpful on many levels. It can help determine the direction of treatment or even identify that treatment should be stopped. You might make a decision to forego a test if it poses a risk to you in disproportion to the benefit of the test result. Sometimes retesting a condition that is thought not likely to change can present the surprise that the condition has improved or no longer exists. Even when treatment is not being given, testing can identify the status of a condition if only to allow a person to project how much time they have to prepare for the end of their life.

Always ask yourself, "What information will the results of this test provide and what value does it have to me?"

Insurance

It is important to understand any insurance policy. For those covered by Medicare, it is important to understand what a benefit period is and how many days of care will be covered while in a facility. Be sure to contact Medicare to verify your current coverage. A benefit period begins the day you enter a Medicare covered facility and ends when you have not received inpatient care in such a facility for 60 days in a row. This period is not based on a calendar year. At this time, Medicare provides full benefits for the first 60 days of inpatient hospital treatment. Should treatment continue, the next 30 days require a copay that may be paid by a secondary insurance policy. After that, up to the next 60 days can be covered as part of a one-time use "lifetime reserve" benefit. Should treatment end before or on the 60th day, no more days can be covered until the patient has had 60 days of no claims. Then the original 60 days of coverage are replenished and can be used. The additional lifetime days are never replenished. In contrast, after fulfilling a three-day inpatient hospital requirement, the first 20 days in a skilled nursing facility are covered by Medicare, after which there is a copay for days 21-100. While you really don't have a choice if you need treatment, it is helpful to know what the parameters of insurance coverage are.

🐞🐞🐞 While a patient has the right to leave a facility at any time, if a patient chooses to leave a facility prior to completion of their treatment plan, they will not be considered officially discharged. If they later return to a facility due to reason that might have been prevented if the treatment plan had been completed, such as a fall, Medicare may deny coverage. Always know the potential consequences of prematurely leaving a facility.

🐞🐞 According to AARP, the Medicare medication "donut hole," the period of time during which medications are not covered, is scheduled to close in 2019.

🐞

Long-Term Care Insurance
Private insurance and Medicare do not cover long-term care. Long-term care is care required due to chronic illness, disabilities or other conditions requiring assistance with ADLs. Private insurance and Medicare may pay some medical expenses but do not pay for daily care. Long-term care insurance (LTCI) is designed to protect your savings and assets by covering some of the cost of long-term care. My parents had LTCI, and it was invaluable. For nearly 16 months, both of my parents required full-time care. We would not have been able to provide both of them the degree of care that they desired without the insurance benefits.

Because we cannot predict the future of our care needs, LTCI policies need to offer flexible options. Policies are designed to cover care in home, in an assisted-living facility or in a nursing home. Additionally, some policies cover care coordination, adult day care, modification of your home for safety and other services.

🐞 Most policies require medical information and an interview to qualify for the policy.

🐞🐞🐞 LTCI policies are not inexpensive. Many people think that they can save the money for long-term care on their own. There are online tools that will determine the expense of an LTCI policy and compare it with how much money would have to be saved to receive the same benefit.

There are several policy features, for which options can be chosen, that affect the cost of an LTCI policy.

- Terms of service: selection of a number of years of coverage, which is then calculated into the number of days covered that can be taken nonconsecutively
- Shared Care policy rider: the option for married couples or partners to share their policy benefits, requiring that both parties have an individual policy
- Elimination period: the number of days you are certified as "eligible for benefits" prior to receiving them, a period which can be waived for in-home care or entirely. The shorter the elimination period, the more expensive the policy. Some policies are based on a one-time elimination period and others require the period for each activation of services.
- Waiver of premium during benefits or after death: allows for waiver of premium payments during activation of benefits.
- Approved providers: Some policies require agencies, registries and independent caregivers to be approved for coverage of their services.
- Inflation protection: selection of percentage of inflation rate of policy benefits

Benefits are requested by initiating a claim. Activation of benefits is based on needed assistance with a predetermined number of ADLs or severe cognitive impairment. An RN approved by the LTCI company will visit the patient and assess their eligibility. If the patient is eligible for benefits and any elimination period has been fulfilled, they will begin filing claims against the policy for services received and be compensated according to the terms of the policy. A patient may improve and no longer need long-term care, and the benefits will be suspended. The benefits may be reactivated at a future time, requiring a reassessment of eligibility.

🐞🐞 This is a very brief explanation of LTCI. Check with an LTCI agent to inquire about current coverage options.

🐞🐞🐞 The most common "mistake" that I see is that people wait too long to initiate a claim for long-term care insurance. They think it is better to save the insurance for when they do not have enough money to pay for care. In reality they may wait so long that they don't live to use their benefits. Policyholders should use their benefits as soon as they are eligible, and allow their personal money to continue to grow. Use your benefits!

Other Considerations
There are issues that must be considered when caring for a senior.

Decisions
Previously I said that my sisters and I gathered information and presented it to our parents so that they could make informed decisions. It was important for them to feel empowered in regard to their own health. That said, a medical crisis can be overwhelming for the patient. While my sisters and I always wanted our parents to make their own decisions, they often looked at us and said, "Well, you think we should do this, don't you?" Even in making their own decisions, they wanted the support of our concurrence.

We presented information to our Dad who had Alzheimer's. Even if he could not make the decision himself, it was important for him to hear the information and to have the right to make a decision even if he only asked us what we thought he should do.

Driving

We want seniors to continue driving as long as they drive safely. Preserving a person's independence is important and it can be difficult to determine when a person's driving is no longer safe. The conversation about whether a person should continue to drive is not easy but it is necessary to prevent injury to the person and other drivers. Before you have that conversation, put yourself in the person's position and imagine having to relinquish your keys, knowing that it means that you will no longer be independent.

With a little searching, it is possible to find organizations that can assist with the process of helping a senior relinquish their driving rights. Today, services like Uber and Lyft are available to provide reasonably priced transportation without requiring that cash or credit cards be carried. Depending on the area in which the senior lives, there may be public transportation geared toward seniors. If the senior is using a wheelchair, there are taxis and vans equipped to allow a person to enter them while in a wheelchair. And, some senior centers and churches offer transportation to seniors.

For those who can continue driving, CarFit (www.car-fit.org), part of the AARP Driver Safety program, offers an educational program that provides seniors the opportunity to check how well their vehicle "fits' them for maximum comfort and safety. This includes checking the driver's ability to see over the steering wheel, their position relative to the air bag, the fit of the seatbelt, proper alignment of the head restraint, access to the gas and brake pedals, position of the mirrors and more. They may also be able to recommend simple adaptive devices such as visor or seat belt extenders, as well as devices which may require an expert's advice such as seat lifts and pedal extenders.

My parents were cooperative. My Dad simply quit driving one day and allowed my Mom to drive them everywhere. I think that he probably had gotten lost and it scared him. With Mom, she wanted to go take her driver's license test for her 91st birthday. Although she did not need to drive, as her family and caregivers were available to transport her, she insisted that she could still drive safely. There was no one contesting that belief. In the end, it came down to the fact that it was just too much work and expense to get her car ready for the test, so she sold it and didn't take the test. Not everyone is so lucky.

Disabled Parking Placard
Parking placards are made available to people with disabilities. The placard allows the operator of the vehicle special privileges regarding the parking of that vehicle. It may be issued as a short-term (90 days), long-term or permanent placard, as well as a permanent license plate. Application for a placard must be submitted with certification of need by a medical doctor. It may also require that the disabled person appear in person at a DMV to complete the application process. If your placard is temporary, you will have to renew it before it expires.

Each state has its own forms and criteria for disabled parking placards. Goggle your state name followed by "disabled parking placard" for information on your state's requirements.

Elder Abuse

> If we do not learn to look after
> and to respect our elderly,
> we will be treated in the same way.
> The quality of a society, I mean of a civilization,
> is also judged on how it treats elderly people
> and by the place it gives them in community life.
> Pope Francis

When I was given the news that my Dad was diagnosed with Alzheimer's, I made a promise to myself that I would protect him and keep him safe at all costs. When he went into skilled rehabilitation and my family was introduced to the need for patient advocacy (see *A Most Meaningful Life,* Chapter 6), I made the verbal promise to my Dad. Proudly I can say with complete assurance that my mom or dad were never abused in their home or in any facility.

Elder Abuse, the taking advantage or mistreatment of seniors 65+, is a significant problem in the United States. It can happen to anyone, anywhere. According to the American Psychological Association, an estimated 2.1 million older Americans become victims on the spectrum of abuse and neglect. It is particularly likely to happen if the person is mentally impaired.

Elder abuse comes in many forms:
- Physical: nonaccidental use of force resulting in pain or injury
- Emotional: degradation, intimidation, humiliation
- Psychological: nonverbal, mental cruelty
- Sexual: nonconsensual contact
- Neglect: failure to provide proper care

- Fraud: misuse of personal checks, credit cards and accounts; stealing, forging and identity theft; and improper use of guardianship or conservatorship
- Exploitation, financial or material: scams
  🐞🐞 The following resources may be helpful in minimizing scams.
  o Contact the Federal Trade Commission to opt out of unsolicited mail, phone calls and email. Google "Federal Trade Commission opt out."
  o Call 888-382-1222 from your phone to opt out of telemarketer calls. You may still receive telemarketing calls from businesses with which you do business, non-profit organizations and political calls.
  o The National Crime Prevention Council provides information regarding safety. www.NCPA.org.
- Abandonment
- The right to control your own life, unless incapacitated

Some neglect is unintentional and caused by family members who, while possibly well-intentioned, are ignorant about proper care. Elder abuse and neglect are not just an assault on a person's quality of life, it often results in premature death.

The actual number of elder-abuse victims is far higher than the estimated 2.1 million, as elder abuse is often not reported. Victims are embarrassed or afraid. The family and friends of victims with dementia who are living in care facilities often do not report the abuse, because they are uninformed about what constitutes abuse, they are absent from the care process, or they are in denial and afraid of finding an alternative.

The movie star Mickey Rooney suffered elder abuse at the hands of his stepson and stepson's wife. He said that he was kept a prisoner in his own home and was threatened, intimidated and harassed. His stepson gained control of his finances, blocked emails and forced him into public performances he did not want to do. The abuse was ongoing, but Rooney was embarrassed and overwhelmed by it. He finally went public with it in 2011. In late 2011, Rooney's stepson and his wife agreed to a settlement for the millions of dollars they had siphoned from Rooney. He was granted court protection from his abusers. In 2014, he appeared before Congress, relaying his story and asking Congress to make elder abuse a specific crime. For an update on elder-abuse legislation, check with your state.

Elder Care Oversight
Determining the care for another person is a big responsibility. And with the statistics on elder abuse, it is clearly very important to identify someone you trust to oversee your care. That is why everyone needs up-to-date, clear and detailed estate planning. (See P*eaceful Endings*, Chapter 2 and the Afterword.) Designating your power of attorneys helps alleviate any question about who has authority to make decisions on your behalf.

There are times when a power of attorney's decisions are called into question. An example has been in the news recently. Tim Conway's family has been in court to determine who will provide the best care for the comedian and actor who was recently diagnosed with dementia. The motives of his wife, who has medical power of attorney, are being questioned in court by Conway's children, who are concerned that their father will not continue to receive the best-possible care. The court has temporarily decided to leave control with Conway's wife, but the children are overseeing the situation with the court's attention. Fortunately, the court system has the authority to resolve estate planning that is contested.

Outings
Outings with seniors, especially if they have medical issues, can present a variety of challenges. For outings with Mom and Dad, we packed a separate day bag for each of them that was always ready.

Each bag contained:
- A copy of their driver's license or state id and insurance cards
- Disabled parking placard
- Devices used to assist with getting in and out of a car
- Chux: can be used to protect any surface including a car seat
- Non-skid mat to step on when getting out of the car
- Nitrile gloves
- Masks
- Gait belt
- Hand wipes
- Hearing aid batteries
- Chip clips: useful in holding a shirt tail up to prevent falling in the toilet
- One-drop toilet deodorizer
- Flashlight
- Garbage bags: for trash and to bag dirty clothes
- Napkins, utensils, straws, condiments
- A small towel to act as a lap napkin
- Umbrella
- A change of clothes

- A spiral notebook, if going to a medical provider appointment

Mom's bag also contained all of her ostomy supplies, in case an appliance change was necessary, extra pads and underwear, and a spare ostomy belt.

Dad's bag also contained individual servings of drink and food thickener for his dysphagia and a ball cap to help keep the sun out of his eyes and his head warm.

For each outing, we packed a small cooler bag with a cold pack inside. We put in water bottles or made fresh thickened drinks for Dad and added snacks in case we got delayed.

If we were going to be out during a medication time, we brought the dosage of medication with us and set a phone alarm to remind us to give it at the proper time. We also brought their purse or wallet, regular eye glasses, sunglasses and a jacket. If they needed to use a walker, they used it to get to the car. In times when they might unexpectedly need additional assistance, we put the transport chair and a chair pad in the trunk of the car as a backup to the walker.

Then we were on our way, prepared for the outing and any delays that might occur.

After an outing, if necessary we cleaned and repacked the bag with any supplies that had been used. We also cleaned the cold pack bag and dumped any unused drinks and perishable snacks. Then we were prepared for the next outing.

Medical Facility Admission
Chapter 6 includes a list of what to bring to a facility to provide comfort and ensure safety when a senior is an inpatient.

Fall prevention
As we age and when we are sick or fall, we are likely to hear, "You're just getting old." Maybe you believe that you are getting old and that falling is a symptom of aging. Falling is not a part of normal aging. But, every 11 seconds an older adult visits the ED for a fall-related injury. According to the National Council on Aging, one in four seniors 65+ will fall annually, often with devastating consequences. Most of those falls are preventable by eliminating hazards in their home. Poor vision, hearing and balance play a major role in falls, and occasionally medication side effects increase the risk of falls. The fear of falling causes seniors to limit mobility, often resulting in isolation and loss of physical fitness.

Regardless of age, several things can be done to reduce your risk of falling. It is important to do the following.
- Make the living space safe by removing items which could cause someone to trip, including throw rugs; creating adequate lighting; and using assistive devices such as bath mats, grab bars, hand rail, a raised toilet seat and a shower bench when necessary.
- Continue to move and to consciously work on improving balance. Exercise programs are an opportunity to both move and improve balance while providing socialization. As we age, the phrase "use it or lose it" is especially true.

- Have vision and hearing tested yearly. The body receives a large portion of its sensory input through the eyes and ears, information that is instrumental in determining balance.
- Discuss medications with a pharmacist to identify any that may increase the risk of falling. It is particularly important if you take multiple medications, as the risk may be increased when they are taken in combination.

You can find more information on preventing falls by Googling "fall prevention."

Preserving Family History and Memories

We were very fortunate that we had a caregiver who offered to create a memory book for her clients. She did so for my parents and created one book that contained their shared history and memories. It seemed fitting as they had been married for nearly 69 years. Because my dad had Alzheimer's, my mom provided the information for my dad's part of the book.

My mom and the caregiver sat for an hour or two every Sunday afternoon for many weeks. They dedicated the time for the caregiver to ask my mom many questions about my parents' history and some of their memories. Once the caregiver was done with typing and formatting the information, my sister and I spent some time researching a few answers that Mom no longer remembered but that were found in a couple of their college year books. The result is an invaluable book, one that I will treasure for the rest of my life.

I cannot recommend highly enough taking the time to preserve your family's history and memories. Interview your loved one before they're gone. Brendon Burchard, high-performance coach, wrote a blog titled just that, "Interview your loved ones before they're gone." In it he suggested 32 questions to ask a person. It is a great place to start and then add your own questions, possibly those specific to your family. To see what Brendon suggested, Google "Brendon Burchard Interview your loved ones before they're gone" or visit http://brendonburchard.tumblr.com/post/98560312858/int erview-your-loved-ones-before-theyre-gone. About half way down the article you will find a link to his interview guide that can be downloaded. You can also find his article and list of questions on facebook: https://www.facebook.com/brendonburchardfan/posts/982 909135076047:0.

Do it before it's too late.

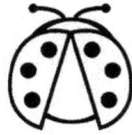

To make a difference in someone's life
you don't have to be
wise, rich, or beautiful.
You just have to be there
when they need you.
Steve Aitchison

Chapter 11

HELPFUL DURABLE EQUIPMENT NONDURABLE EQUIPMENT AND SUPPLIES ...
life made easier

When my sisters and I were caregivers for my parents, we often felt the need for equipment or supplies to make certain activities easier for my parents and for us. We had no idea what equipment and supplies were available, or whether my parents' insurance plans would cover the cost. The answer to the coverage question is that some items were covered, while others were not. For example, insurance would pay for a standard hospital bed if a physician's prescription was submitted. The insurance plan would not cover the additional cost for a bed with an electronic mechanism to raise and lower it. My mom was willing to pay the additional expense because it would be easier for the in-home caregivers. Prior to having in-home caregivers, we were really on our own to investigate what equipment and supplies were available or useful. Experienced caregivers are a great resource for practical solutions to problems. In addition, when my parents started qualifying for in-home health services, additional equipment and supplies were available for coverage under their insurance plans.

Equipment can be a double-edged sword. It can preserve independence or provide respite for a caregiving spouse, but it can also promote immobility and resultant loss of muscle mass. We always encouraged our parents to do as much as possible for themselves in order to keep their strength, as well as large and small motor skills. Some days they would be able to use a walker and others they required a transport chair, but the preference was always that they walk as much as possible. The balance in the use of equipment is between necessity and convenience. Necessity is not optional but convenience should be occasional.

Medical Equipment and Supplies
There are different classifications for equipment and supplies.

Durable medical equipment is equipment that:
- Will withstand repeated use
- Serves a medical purpose and is not useful in the absence of medical need
- Is appropriate for use in the home
- Is expected to last for three years or more

This includes items such as hospital beds, wheel chairs, walkers and portable oxygen equipment.

Nondurable medical equipment and supplies include equipment such as over-the-bed tray tables and transfer benches. Supplies are disposable medical and nonmedical items, including ostomy supplies, bed pads and gloves.

There are many sources of durable medical equipment, nondurable medical equipment and supplies. And, there are varying criteria that determine whether or not an insurance plan will cover them and whether a prescription from a physician is required. In addition, Medicare and Medicaid require that equipment and many supplies be acquired from their approved suppliers. Under Medicare and Medicaid, some supplies are covered with a physician's prescription and others are covered only if the supplies are for use by home-health providers. Some nonprofits and senior centers rent or loan durable equipment. Call your local Area Agency on Aging for assistance. Google: "find local Area Agency on Aging" followed by your zipcode or county and state or visit http://www.n4a.org. Otherwise, call your county and ask to be directed to the senior services department. Finally, it is an option to purchase equipment and supplies out of pocket.

I suggest asking every medical professional what equipment and supplies they find helpful and would recommend for your specific situation. One of the most helpful supplies was suggested to us in a passing remark made by a hospital transportation volunteer as he wheeled my mom to a radiology appointment. Ask everyone and listen.

Assistance, Safety, Comfort and Convenience
There are many items that can be helpful in assisting with ADLs, promoting a patient's safety, providing comfort and increasing convenience. Following are the items my family found helpful. Your situation may warrant different items, and you will likely find what you need.

Functional Mobility or Transferring
These are items that assist with walking and getting into and out of a bed or a chair.
You can use the bolded and italicized names below in a Google search to find these items.

- Hospital beds
  A hospital bed is helpful in not only assisting the patient with getting in and out of bed, but also assists the

203

caregiver by not requiring them to bend over the bed. The bed is delivered with a mattress. It is sometimes an air mattress and others times a solid mattress.

The standard bed has a hand crank for raising and lowering the bed, as well as raising and lowering the head and foot of the bed. For an additional cost to the patient, a hospital bed can include an electric mechanism with a remote control.

🐞🐞 Most hospital beds require *extra-long sheets*. They generally are available at Target for sale to college students. Pretty sheets help the patient feel good. If possible, purchase a couple of sets to allow time for changing and washing them.

🐞🐞🐞 We learned that during the first year, while Medicare was paying for the bed, the supplier considered the hospital bed rented, and therefore if it were no longer needed during the first year, we had to return it. After a year, the hospital bed became our property.

o   Additional bed padding
    If the patient will be in a bed more than a regular sleep cycle, consider adding something to reduce pressure resulting in bed sores. Either an *alternating air pressure mattress* (may be covered by insurance) or a foam *mattress topper* (sometimes called an egg crate and not usually covered by insurance but inexpensive) can be used. My mom had arthritis, and found that the air mattresses and pads caused her pain. Therefore, we used a foam topper on her bed.

🐞🐞 Some facilities offered the use of a mattress topper, but it could take days to receive it. They were not available in other facilities. We always brought our own twin mattress topper to the facilities.

o   Waterproof sheets and pads
    Using a **mattress protector** or **waterproof sheet** and/or **waterproof bed pads** can minimize laundry and save your mattress from damage. The pads can also be placed on top of the sheets.

o   Transfer sheet
    A transfer sheet is a **top bedsheet** that is laid across the width of the bed, at about hip level, and folded to a width of about 30 inches. It is placed on top of the bottom sheet and under any protective products such as pads. It is used to move the patient while in bed.

o   Styrofoam roller
    Placing a **styrofoam circle roller** (6" diameter x 36") under the sheet and at the end of the bed can prevent the sheets from pulling on the patient's toes and causing numbness and pain. It also allows for some air flow at the end of the bed. The rollers can even be used at the sides of the bed, under the sheets, to create a **bed bumper** which prevents the patient from rolling or falling out of bed.

    A small roller, or a rolled hand towel, placed under the ankles can prevent the heels from becoming irritated or sore from constant pressure while in bed.

o Bed tray table
While in bed, *a bed tray table or bedside table* is useful while doing activities such as eating, reading and writing. Some trays hang over the bed and are attached to wheels that go under the bed. Other trays are foldable and sit on the bed. Insurance may cover some trays and not others.

o Bed rail
Bed rails come in multiple lengths. After my dad was injured when he fell out of bed and hit his face on his nightstand, my family used a ¼ length bedrail to ensure that it would not happen again. The ¼ length rail was also helpful in assisting my dad in sitting up from bed and swinging his legs over the side. This rail had pockets on the outside in which we could store tissues. At another time, we used a single full-length rail to prevent my dad from getting out of bed on the side opposite his walker. In some medical care facilities, a full-length bedrail is considered a restraint and is not allowed. In others, they allow a bedrail on only one side of the bed at a time.

🐞🐞 Every facility in which my parents stayed provided *nonskid socks*, which we then took home. We found it helpful to tie the socks to the end of the bed so that we could always find them.

- Lift
For those who cannot assist with transferring, especially those who are wheelchair bound, there are lifts that can assist a caregiver with moving the patient.

- Seat-lifting assistance
  While a *reclining chair* offers benefits, such as elevating legs, some offer additional assistance with rising out of the chair. There are also *seat assist or stand assist* devices that can be placed in an existing chair and gives the patient a boost when rising to stand.

- Transfer slide
  This is a board with a swivel sliding seat that allow a person to transfer between a bed, wheelchair, commode, shower seat or car and back again. It eliminates the need to be lifted by another person.

- Wheelchairs
  The traditional *wheelchair* is a substantial, often heavy, chair with wheels. If a patient is going to spend much time in the wheelchair, the traditional style is the most supportive. It is also the heaviest, sometimes around 40 pounds, to lift in and out of a vehicle. There are also motorized wheelchairs that provide independence for those who navigate primarily indoors. An alternative is the *transport chair*, a light weight wheelchair weighing around 25 pounds with a smaller profile, particularly helpful for those who need only occasional assistance. With either product, *a chair pad* is helpful in providing comfort.

- Mobility Scooter
  A scooter is a mobility option for those who may want to maneuver outdoors as well as indoors, and can transfer themselves on and off of the scooter. It may be an option for someone who wants the independence of going to the local store but no longer drives and can't walk long distances.

- Walkers

  Several different types of **walkers** are available. Some walkers include a seat, which is helpful when the patient is away from home and becomes fatigued. An upright walker allows the person to stand upright when using the walker, supporting the person under their elbows therefore eliminating the slight bend required when using a traditional walker. We attached a cloth bag to the front of the walker frame to hold eye glasses, tissues, a book and other items.

- Canes

  Canes are used for support when one leg is not fully supportive. They are made of several materials and come in varieties such as adjustable and collapsible. The handle may be purely functional or decorative to add a little personality to the equipment.

- Gait belts

  A **gait belt** is a strap that is used to assist a patient while walking. The belt is worn around the patient's waist and provides a means by which the caregiver can provide support to the patient when walking or transferring positions. Most facilities have a gait belt available for use with each new patient. It is an invaluable safety tool **when used properly**. When leaving a facility in which a gait belt was used, ask if you can take the belt with you. If you have in-home health services, they will provide a gait belt. Our caregivers and our family members sometimes used the gait belt when we no longer had in-home health services and we were at home providing care for our parents.

🐞🐞 Be sure to be trained by a professional on the correct and safe use of a gait belt.

🐞🐞🐞 **Never** use a regular belt instead of a gait belt. Regular belts are attached to clothing, usually pants, and will pull that clothing up when lifted. Also, regular belts are not designed to bear the weight of a person.

Bathing/Showering

Not only are bathing and showering difficult, they can be very hazardous. Assistance with the physical activities of bathing and showering may be covered by insurance, but safety devices are likely not.

- Grab bars
  Grab bars are specifically designed to assist with the transfer in and out of a shower or tub, or on and off of a toilet. They should be placed where a person needs stability, including inside a shower and strategically near a bath tub. Be sure that a grab bar placed near the tub is positioned low enough to be of assistance in rising from the tub. They should also be added to the wall near a toilet.

  🐞🐞🐞 Towel bars and shower rods **are not substitutes** for grab bars and it would be dangerous to used them as such. Their installation, strength and intended purpose are very different than that of grab bars.

  🐞🐞🐞 Be sure that the grab bars are professionally installed.

- Benches

  There are many types of **bath benches.** Some have adjustable legs for varying heights. Benches are placed in the shower or tub and allow the patient to safely sit. **Transfer benches** help a patient safely "slide" over a tub side or a shower lip and often have backs on them.

  👀👀 While not a bench, it is important to know that there is a **bath lift** on which a patient sits and can be lowered into and raised out of a tub.

- Nonslip shower and tub surface

  There are **nonslip shower stick-on decals**, but I have found **Tub Grip Clear anti-slip bathroom coating by Grip-It** to be the most reliable product. I do **not** recommend using a suction bath mat because if they are not solidly suctioned to the tub they will slip.

- Removable showerhead

  A **hand-held removable showerhead**, mounted at an easily reachable height, allows it to be used as a showerhead or hand-held sprayer.

- Single-lever faucets

  Faucets with knobs are difficult for many people to turn and also require the coordination of both cold and hot water. A **single-lever faucet** provides ease of use and temperature control

- Dispensers for products

  The use of **shower dispensers** for shampoo, conditioner, and body soap avoid the lifting and the need to pick up an item that has fallen onto the shower floor.

- Container for hearing aids
  Having a container for storage of hearing aids in the shower helped to remind us to remove them prior to starting the water. A sturdy plastic bag can be used.

- Supplies for a bed bath
  These include **plastic wash basins** for water (one for wash water and one for rinse water), several wash cloths and *pure soap.* Antibacterial soap is not as effective. We used *Ivory* or ***Dr. Bronner's Pure Castille*** soap and large bath towels.

Toileting
Toileting can be difficult as it requires getting on and off the toilet as well as cleaning oneself.

- Toilet safety rails
  I mentioned grab bars above. The addition of **toilet safety rails** can greatly assist with lowering to and rising from the toilet.

- Toilet seat riser
  A ***toilet seat riser*** is placed on top of the actual toilet seat to assist when the toilet is too low for the patient.

  🐞🐞 17" "comfort height" toilets are now available.

- Specimen collector for urine or stool
  Also known as a "toilet hat", a ***specimen collector*** is useful to catch samples for testing, as well as to measure urine output. The hat is placed under the toilet seat. ***Specimen cups or containers*** are handy to have in the event that a physician orders a urinalysis and the patient cannot leave home.

- Over the toilet shelf
  An **over-the-toilet storage shelf or organizer** allows for easy access to supplies necessary for toileting such as: a baby wipe warmer with wipes, barrier cream or wipes, bleach water for cleanups and any special items such as those needed for colostomy care. It can be a single shelf or a multi-shelf unit.

- Commode
  Once a person can no longer use the toilet in the bathroom, a **bedside commode** may be necessary. Consider the way in which the bucket is accessible. Some buckets have lids. I strongly recommend placing a **commode mat** under the commode for easy cleanup. Some mats are fiber and others are a washable hard surface. 👀 👀 We used an **office desk mat**. Be sure than any mat is securely placed under the commode.

- Bedpan
  There are different kinds of **bedpans**. Some are metal, others plastic. They can be thick or low profile and contoured. Finding one that the person can effectively use is important. If a bedpan has been used during a stay in a facility, you can take it home.

  👀 👀 We always placed a disposable absorbent material in the bedpan to soak up urine and to prevent spills when removing the pan. There are small pads that are good for this purpose. You could also use a washable cloth diaper.

- Urinal
  Use of a **urinal** can reduce visits to the bathroom, especially at night.

212

- Disposable underwear
  Depends is one brand of **disposable or incontinence underwear**. There are thicker products which are used for incontinence and lower-profile products for protection from accidents. There are products that provide more protection for overnight, as well as liners that can be added to the products to increase protection. During the night, it is sometimes possible to change the liner without having to change the entire undergarment. For those who cannot get out of bed, adult "tabbed" underwear, unflatteringly called adult diapers, are available. A skilled caregiver can change the tabbed underwear with the person in bed.

  👀 👀 While a valuable and often necessary product, disposable underwear can trap heat and result in heat rash. Cleaning the skin, letting it dry and dusting antifungal powder, _not baby powder_, will help to keep the skin clear. Also, it is important to check the undergarment frequently so that it is changed as soon as it is soiled.

- A small space heater
  This kept the bathroom toasty warm without having to heat the entire home.

- Odor eliminator
  This is one of the most valuable products that I found and used. It is sometimes difficult to assist another person with toileting because of the smell. Products like **One Drop by Sawaday** are a lifesaver. Literally one drop in the toilet or commode prior to use and there was virtually no smell. If we were not collecting urine or fecal samples, we put clean water and a drop in the commode

213

bucket immediately after cleaning it, so that it was ready for the next use. Also, breathing through your mouth helps.

Personal Hygiene, Grooming and Dressing
(brushing/combing hair, oral care)

- Personal cleansing washcloths
  These are large adult disposable washcloths that are useful for quick freshening up when a full bath is not possible.

- Hand wipes
  Wet Ones (antibacterial) and Purell sanitizing wipes are invaluable when in public.

- Baby wipes
  Be sure you know if the wipes are flushable or not. *Non-flushable wipes go in the trash only*. Be sure they do not contain alcohol which can sting the skin.

- Baby-Wipe Warmer
  Although it was not recommended by the baby-wipe warmer companies to place wipes other than baby wipes in the warmer, we placed a couple of baby wipes along with a couple of barrier wipes in the baby-wipe warmer so that they would not be cold when we used them.

- Moisture-barrier products
  There are many products available to provide moisture-barrier skin protection, specifically from urine and feces. There are wipes and creams. I preferred Sage barrier wipes.

- Diaper rash and wound-protection cream
  These products are more substantial than barrier products. They are usually thick creams, pastes or ointments that form a visible layer of protection. I preferred Boudreaux's Butt Paste.

  👀 👀 Butt Paste is initially applied in a thick layer. Each time cleaning is needed, the top layer is "scraped" off, leaving the unsoiled protective layer on the skin. When the final layer is removed, a new thick layer is applied.

- Antifungal powder
  Desenex powder helps prevent and treat heat rash wherever skin touches other skin, especially in the armpits, leg joints and skin folds.

- Antibiotic, cortisone and hemorrhoid creams
  Having these on hand eliminated an emergency run to the store.

- Mouth sponges, oral swabs
  Useful when a person cannot sit up to brush their teeth

- Foot/hand cream and body lotion
  Help prevent dry skin

- Artificial tears, saline nasal spray, lip balm

- Small or travel-size toothpaste
  Provided ease of use, as well as reduced waste when the lid was not closed properly

Self-Feeding

- Smaller eating utensils
  Easier for the patient to lift and encourage smaller, safer bites of food

- Small, light-weight drinking cups
  Easier for patient to lift and minimizes spills

- A nonslip plate mat
  Helps to keep a meal plate in place

- Nice large napkins and decorative dishes
  Makes the eating experience more enjoyable. The use of **napkin clips (alligator clips)** with fabric napkins eliminates the use of bibs.

Safety

- Monitors and alarms
  - Bed or floor-mat alarm
    A bed alarm sounds when a person has gotten out of bed and removed their weight from the bed mat. A floor mat alarms when pressure is applied to the mat, as when a person stands on it.

  - Motion alarm
    Indicates that the person is moving. We initially used it to let us know that my dad was opening the bedroom door. We later repositioned it to notify us that he was getting out of bed. Door alarms are also available. We found that the motion alarm was most versatile.

o Motion-activated light
   Can be used to turn on a light as a patient moves past
   it. It is especially useful in lighting the way from a
   bedroom to a bathroom.

o Audio monitor
   A baby monitor is useful in monitoring a patient
   when they are in another room. The patient can use
   it to call for assistance and/or it allows a caregiver to
   hear noise made when a patient wakes up during the
   night.

o Video baby monitor
   Can be used to visually monitor the patient from
   another room. We did not find a use for this.

o Call button
   Can be kept with the patient and used to notify
   caregivers that the patient needs assistance. This was
   helpful in the middle of the night as well as when our
   parents were ready for assistance after using the toilet
   or commode. Using a **caregiver pager with call
   buttons** *is one option*. We placed a **steel silver hand
   bell** near Mom's pillow and one by the commode.

o Smoke and carbon monoxide alarms
   Smoke alarms should be on every floor, inside of
   every bedroom and in the basement A carbon
   monoxide detector should be on every floor, 5 feet
   from the ground. They should also be near a gas
   furnace and a gas clothes dryer.

o Toilet Alarm
   Notifies a caregiver that a toilet has not properly
   flushed. There are **water-sensor alarms** for the floor

217

which may work well if someone is always in the home. We used a more sophisticated **_toilet alarm_** that not only sensed the water level in the tank and bowl, but also shut the water off if the water level had risen too high.

- Phone for seniors
  Landline and mobile phones offer options that include easier menus and larger buttons, and others that work well with hearing aids. Jitterbug is one of many options and offers both a flip phone and a smart phone.

- Video chat
  Offered in different ways and promotes connection with family and friends. ViewClix smart frame (www.ViewClix.com) offers easy access to shared pictures and videos and video calling. GrandPad (www.GrandPad.NET) is a tablet designed for seniors offering calling, email, shared photos, a camera, music and much more. GrandPad operates on a data plan to avoid the need for a WIFI connection. The Wow! Computer (www.MyWowComputer.com) is a simple to use computer designed especially for seniors that offers functions similar to GrandPad but requires an Internet connection.

Starting with the word "seniors", Google any of the following to find devices offering the features above: smart frame, shared photos, video calling, tablet or computer. Add "simple to use" to any of the Google searches.

- Hearing: Sonic cloud
  For those with hearing loss, SonicCloud is an app that facilitates hearing of phone calls, video, movies, TV shows and music. Visit www.SonicCloud.com.

- Monitoring
  Everyday there are more applications available to assist caregivers and families in monitoring the care of their seniors. They monitor everything from movement to medications and offer coordination of caregivers. Senior-based businesses such as AARP and A Place for Mom often do reviews of the most current apps available. Examples of apps are Caring Village, CareZone, Lotsa Helping Hands and Caringbridge, each offering a variety of benefits. Googling "caregiver monitoring apps" will give you a start to finding the apps that work on smartphones and tablets.

- Medical alert device
  There are many medical alert devices, also known as personal emergency response systems (PERS). A PERS device can be used to alert a central monitoring system when assistance is needed. The need for assistance can be due to a medical emergency or the result of a fall, or the device can be used to notify someone that the person is locked out of their home, lost or feels unsafe. It can also be used in the case of fire or home invasion. Some systems offer a necklace or bracelet that can be worn. Some devices require the use of a landline connection and will not work outside of the home. Others work off of mobile connection and can be used while away from home, including while traveling. Following are a few options that offer PERS services:

Life Alert (www.LifeAlert.com),
Lively mobile (www.Livelydirect.com) and
MobileHelp (www.mobilehelp.com)
To find more options, Google "mobile medical alert."

Monitoring Vitals
- Digital thermometers
  Easiest to use and different types can be used orally, in the ear, on the forehead or rectally.

- A watch or a clock with a second hand
  Used for manually checking a pulse and respirations.

- A Pulse oximeter
  Checks pulse and oxygen level. It is sometimes called a pulseox.

- A blood-pressure cuff and stethoscope
  Should be used only by a healthcare professional to check blood pressure. Others can use a digital monitor.

  👀👀 As a patient ages bps taken digitally may be inaccurate. If a bp does not seem correct, have a healthcare professional verify it using the manual method.

- Bathroom scale

First Aid
- First-aid supplies
  There are many kits available that offer a variety of antiseptic towelettes, first-aid cream, various sizes of bandages, gauze, burn relief, insect-sting relief, first-aid tape, moleskin squares, an instant cold compress and

tweezers. In addition, you may want cortisone cream, liquid bandage and products to stop bleeds.

- For bleeding
  Be sure that any product, such as WoundSeal powder, is safe for a person on blood thinners. There are nose plugs and strips too.

- Tampons
  Good for absorbing blood, particularly from a nose bleeds.

- Teabags
  An alternative to gauze for absorbing blood, particularly in the mouth.

- Arnica and Hemp Oil
  Arnica, an herb used to help heal inflamed or bruised skin and relieve aches, found in Arnicare gel by Boiron and hemp oil in Comfort Balm by Restorative Botanicals are both helpful to reduce aches and pains.

Other Supplies
- Disposable, absorbent and washable underpads
  Disposable pads are useful in protecting bedding, chairs and car seats. Washable underpads are thicker and sturdier. Both come in multiple sizes. The washable pads come in a long length which helps to line a bed. Disposable underpads come in varying qualities depending on the brand. I suggest ordering a small quantity at first to see what the quality is. We used several sizes of both types of underpads.

👀👀 The original disposable and absorbent pads were called chux, as they were literally chucked into the garbage. Chux is now synonymous with disposable absorbent underpads, which are typically blue but sometimes now green.

- Gloves
  Must be worn whenever exposure to bodily fluids is possible. Many people have latex allergies therefore, we used *nitrile gloves*. We also chose to use powder-free gloves. We had a variety of caregiver hand sizes and had to purchase multiple sizes. I used two sizes of gloves depending on the kind of work I was doing. If the work required fine skill I had to wear a tighter glove. If not, I preferred to wear a glove that was looser to allow airflow.

- Face masks
  Used to protect both the caregivers and the patient.

- A nonslip mat:
  Placed on the ground when the patient is stepping out of a car to prevent slipping, especially on ice.

Organization and Setup
- Privacy screens
  Help the patient to feel that their privacy is protected. When a bedroom was set up for my mom in the dining room, we purchased privacy screens so that others in the home could not look into her bedroom space.

- Shelves or dresser
  For organization and easy access storage. In one instance we used a baby changing table.

- Portable table
A ***portable table*** is useful for setting up supplies prior to a procedure, such as changing an ostomy appliance.

- Swing-arm lamp
A swing-arm lamp is invaluable if you will be doing procedures such as changing an ostomy appliance or giving a shot. Proper lighting is critical.

- A small three-tier wire rolling cart
Used to roll supplies to the bed, commode or any other place where they are needed. This was helpful in organizing my mom's ostomy supplies and making them easily accessible.

- Small storage bins
Used to keep like items together, can be stacked on shelves for easy access.

- Paper towels

- Garbage bags
All sizes - small, medium, large and kitchen

- Lysol wipes
For everyday cleanup of counters and toilets.

- Bleach
Used for the most extensive cleaning and sanitization. Bleach kills many bacteria that other products do not. Neither Lysol nor regular Clorox wipes have bleach in them. ***Clorox Healthcare bleach germicidal wipes*** do have bleach, but are expensive. Bleach mixed with water at a 1:9 ratio (one-part bleach to nine-parts of water)

maintains its sanitizing potency for about 24 hours. Bleach mixed at 1:3 (one-part bleach to three-parts water) will remain effective for about a week.

- Ammonia
Adding ammonia to a load of laundry, helps to remove the odors of urine and sweat. <u>Do not inhale vapors</u>.

🐞🐞🐞 **Never use or mix bleach and ammonia** together as it results in toxic vapors that may result in the need for medical attention.

- <u>Hydrogen peroxide</u>
Not only is this used for cleaning minor cuts and scrapes, it is powerful at removing blood from fabrics, including carpet, by dabbing and then blotting it.

- <u>Odor eliminating room spray</u>
Find a spray with as little scent as possible. Many people are allergic to fragrances.

- <u>Office supplies</u>
Scissors, paper, pens, sticky note pads and spiral notebooks

Where to Get Equipment and Supplies
There were many items that my family purchased out of pocket because they were either necessary or useful and not covered by insurance. I always tried to find the best source for each item as the prices varied significantly.

Costco, Walgreens and Amazon offered most items but prices varied. The Internet proved invaluable in allowing me to search for items and compare prices. Googling "in home medical supplies" as well as a specific item's name, such as "transport chair," brought up many online options for purchases. Some items were available only from their manufacturer's website. In addition to pricing I also considered availability, delivery time and cost of shipping. I always reverified the pricing prior to making the next purchase as items often went on sale.

🐞🐞 Amazon often offered the best prices. Their Prime subscription saved us a lot of money on shipping when we did not have a local source. Costco consistently had the best price on Depends underwear and nitrile gloves, and the barrier wipes we liked could only be purchased from the manufacturer Sage.

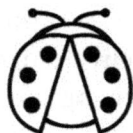

A physician once said,
"The best medicine for humans is love."
Someone asked,
"What if it doesn't work?"
He smiled and said,
"Increase the dose."
Unknown

Chapter 12

DEALING WITH SPECIFIC
MEDICAL ISSUES ...
survival tips

Many times while caring for my parents, my sisters and I found ourselves in a new situation with little direction or proper training. In most cases, we did not understand our options. In the case of the clostridium difficile bacteria, we did not understand the potentially life-threatening severity. We had to understand my parents' medical issues in order to assist with them and to speak with medical providers about them. During one emergency, I was sitting in the front seat of the ambulance while the paramedics provided care for my mom prior to transportation to the ED. The paramedics kept asking my mom medical history questions which I had to answer. At one point I heard, "So, how long have you been an RN?" I did not respond at first but later realized that the question had been addressed to me. I responded that I was not.

This section details my experience with the topics that follow. Although this information was obtained from conversations with many medical professionals, I recommend that you seek the advice of a medical professional in regard to your specific situation.

Cellulitis
Dad had knee surgery and was medically doing well. It's a long story (see *A Most Meaningful Life*, Chapter 6), but after being improperly medicated and overmedicated, he ended

up in skilled rehabilitation. During the first week he began to retain a lot of fluid in his legs. He was given diuretics but the swelling increased. Soon his legs began to look infected, and the skin began to literally weep. He had cellulitis as a result of the ongoing swelling in his legs.

What is it?
Cellulitis is a bacterial skin infection involving the inner layers of the skin. The infection causes swelling and redness and can make the skin feel hot and tender.

How is it treated?
Treatment of the infection requires antibiotics. Reduction of the swelling causing the cellulitis involved elevating Dad's legs and having Dad wear Ted hose, which are compression socks.

👀 👀 👀 The Ted hose were extremely tight and occasionally the nails of the person putting them on Dad would scratch him and pose an additional infection risk. One day an RN was assigned to put the Ted hose on Dad, and she asked why Ted hose were being used instead of putting an Ace bandage on his legs. We did not know the answer, but the Ace bandages were much more comfortable than the Ted hose, and they eliminated the risk of infections caused by scratches.

👀 👀 👀 Eliminating the excess liquid stored in Dad's very swollen legs was paramount to him recovering from cellulitis. Although Dad's legs were elevated while he was in bed, my family felt that a recliner would allow him to be upright during the day with his legs elevated. The facility did not have recliner chairs so we rented one, at our own expense, from a medical supply company. We ordered the chair and had it delivered to the facility. Within 10 days Dad had lost 40 pounds of fluid, his legs were not swollen and the cellulitis infection was healing.

🐞 🐞 🐞 With the elimination of 40 pounds of fluid, Dad had to go to the bathroom very frequently. The medical providers at the facility wanted Dad to use a Foley catheter. We said "No," as it would likely result in a UTI, and that we would be responsible for taking him to the bathroom

🐞

Clostridium Difficile: C. diff

Mom's first medical crisis included several life-threatening conditions, one of which was a perforated colon. With a weakened immune system and the prevalence of bacteria on hospital surfaces, she soon had uncontrollable diarrhea caused by C. diff. Mom was treated for C. diff and re-hospitalized three more times before beating the infection. For the six months during which mom was symptomatic, my family was challenged to prevent her from recontamination and to protect our dad, seven caregivers and our many family members and friends who visited from contamination. Not one person was contaminated, and even Mom's medical professionals were impressed with and surprised by our success.

What is it?

C. diff is a spore-forming bacterium that is found in the environment including the soil, air, food products, and animal and human waste. It can cause severe diarrhea and serious intestinal conditions.

How do you get it?
There are about 1 trillion bacteria in the intestines. Good bacteria help keep the bad bacteria in check. Antibiotics are used to kill bad bacteria but also kill some of the helpful good bacteria. At some point the good bacteria can no longer keep the bad bacteria in check, and the person becomes symptomatic. Some healthy people carry the bacteria and don't have ill effects, as their immune systems are strong and their intestines populated with good bacteria to counteract the bad.

C. diff is considered to be very contagious. The bacteria and spores are found in feces and are spread person-to-person by touch or by direct contact with contaminated surfaces or items when hands are not washed properly.

The illness typically affects older adults in hospitals or long-term care facilities, usually affecting those with weakened immune systems who are being treated with antibiotics or taking proton pump inhibitors. It accounts for 20% of cases of antibiotic-associated diarrhea. Because C. diff is resistant to most common cleaners and it can survive on surfaces for up to five months, C. diff is present on many surfaces in medical facilities.

How do you know you have it?
The main symptom is severe and frequent diarrhea. The presence of C. diff is determined through a stool test.

🐞🐞🐞 My family found that C. diff had a very distinct, pungent smell that each of us described slightly differently. We were able to identify the presence of C. diff by its odor. When I asked an RN about this ability, she said that a group of RNs had been polled to see if they could identify C. diff by smell, and that the results showed that they could not. My family however, could identify it with great accuracy just by the smell.

Why is it so dangerous?
According to *Contagion*, a news resource covering all areas of infectious disease, C. diff was the cause of 450,000 infections and 29,000 deaths in the United States in 2015. Recurrent C. diff doubles the chances of hospital re-admission. For those over 65 years of age, accounting for 2/3rds of the cases of C. diff, morbidity and mortality rates are particularly high. If untreated, C. diff can quickly result in:

- Dehydration
- Kidney failure
- Colitis
- Toxicity
- Perforation of the colon
- Death

How it is treated?
There are two aspects to treatment
1. Treating the infection
    C. diff is receptive to antibiotic treatment, which seems counterintuitive because C. diff is often the result of antibiotic use. The antibiotics that cause C. diff are different than those that treat it. The usual course of treatment is to first treat it with Flagyl (metronidazole). Based on the results of a course of Flagyl, intravenous Vancomycin may either be added to the treatment or used to replace Flagyl. After 10 days or when the stool has returned to a soft form, a six-week cycle of treatment with oral Vancomycin begins. If relapse occurs and Vancomycin is determined to be ineffective, a 10-day

course of Dificid (fidaxomicin) may be prescribed. Taking probiotics is recommended to repopulate the good bacteria in the gut. If a relapse of C. diff continues, a fecal transplant may be discussed.

🐞🐞🐞 At the time that Mom had C. diff, Dificid was a new and very expensive medication. Because Flagyl and Vancomycin were the standard treatments for C. diff, Mom's infectious disease specialist had to contact Medicare to justify coverage of the new, costlier drug.

2. Preventing recontamination
   C. diff is resistant to the most common surface disinfectants. Alcohol, including antibacterial hand wash, does not kill it. Bleach is the only cleaner that can kill it. Pure soap, as opposed to anti-bacterial soap, is thought to be effective in helping to wash the bacteria off of the skin. In order to prevent contamination, as soon as it is suspected that a patient has C. diff, contact precautions are activated: quarantine in a private room with the required use of isolation gowns and gloves for all entering the room. Additional soap-based hand wash is brought into the room to be used instead of the antibacterial soap that is usually used. Use of the bathroom is reserved only for the patient and all items that come into contact with the patient are either properly disposed of or sterilized.

What We Did to Prevent Contamination with C. diff
My family took every precaution, both at medical facilities and at home, to prevent contamination with C. diff. We created a protocol that we documented and with which compliance was required of everyone who entered my

parents' home. Our protocol has been successfully used by others.

- First and foremost, from the first diagnosis of my mom having C. diff, *I completely stopped touching my face with my hands, as did Mom and others.* I used disposable facial wipes and a disposable cup for water when brushing my teeth. This was true for more than six months past Mom's recovery from C. diff.

- Items that were used in my mom's hospital room prior to the initial diagnosis, such as blankets we brought from home, were properly handled. All items were bagged and sealed prior to being bought home. *Items that could not be bleached had to be washed in hot water and dried on a hot setting.* If the item could be, then the item was cleaned. If not, it was kept sealed for 6 months prior to reopening and cleaning.

- 🐞🐞🐞 It was critical for my family to understand the difference among cleaning products. *C. Diff is only killed by bleach.* Lysol wipes and Clorox Disinfecting Wipes **do not** contain bleach and therefore do not kill C. diff. **Only Clorox Healthcare Bleach Germicidal wipes or cleaner or a bleach and water solution will kill C. diff.** We used both the Clorox germicidal products or a solution of bleach and water. We used a spray bottle to dispense the solution. A solution of 1-part bleach to 9 parts water can be used for 24 hours before being replaced. A solution of 1-part bleach to 4 parts water can be used for up to a week.

- *We no longer used anti-bacterial hand soap.* Instead we used only pure soap such as Ivory traditional bar soap or Dr. Bronner's Castille soap.

- Whether at home or in a facility, *we cleaned every surface and item daily*: the bedrails, bedside tables, phone, remote controls and anything that my mom could touch. At home *the toilet or commode was cleaned with every use.* Door handles and any surfaces that multiple people might touch, such as the refrigerator door, were cleaned more frequently.

- While C. diff was active, Mom used a commode instead of the bathroom she usually shared with Dad. We could not take the chance that Dad would be contaminated. When Mom had to use the commode, she wore gloves, as did anyone assisting. Afterward, everyone's hands were washed with warm water and soap and the commode was disinfected. All disposable items that were touched during the process were bagged and disposed of.

- *Mom was given warm soapy towels* to wash her hands before each meal and throughout the day.

- *Everyone who entered my parents' home, including caregivers and family members, were required to wash their hands* both upon entry and exit.

- *We avoided any unnecessary use of antibiotic*s.

- *Whenever we entered any medical facility, we avoided touching any surface without wearing gloves.*

Dysphagia

While Dad was in skilled rehabilitation after knee surgery, the speech therapist heard a gurgling in his throat and observed him continually clearing his throat. She was concerned and ordered a test to identify whether he was aspirating fluid into his lungs. The test indicated that the mechanism that prevents food and fluid from aspirating into the lungs was not always working properly, putting him at risk for aspiration, a condition called dysphagia. With this diagnosis, we were told that in the future all of Dad's meals and drinks had to be prepared so that they were "pudding thick." The first meal arrived and looked like three piles of oatmeal, all the same color and consistency. It was unappetizing to Dad, and he didn't want to eat it. I would not have wanted to either. The next night Dad looked at his plate and asked, "What is that?" I don't lie, and therefore I made my best guess and said "stew," but I had no idea. Eating had always been one of Dad's pleasures, and my family decided that once we had Dad home, we had to do better.

In the beginning, making meals and drinks for dad was a challenge. Again, with no one to provide direction, we made a lot of less than successful attempts. With a constant search for new and better products, we were able to find products that allowed us to prepare meals and drinks that Dad enjoyed.

What is it?

Dysphagia is any problem with swallowing. Many of these problems can lead to aspiration, which means that food or fluids go into the lungs instead of the stomach.

It can happen as the mechanism fails and it is sometimes a temporary post-surgical complication. It is identified when someone has trouble swallowing or sometimes when a speech therapist hears that fluid is not being cleared from the throat. Various techniques used to identify dysphagia during a process called a swallow test. During the test the patient drinks liquids of differing thicknesses. Images are recorded to monitor the swallowing process and identify any malfunctions.

How is it treated?
In some cases, speech therapy can help. In most cases a change to the consistency of food and drinks is required. There may be other treatments dependent on the exact cause of the malfunction.

Food and Drink Categories
At the time Dad was diagnosed with dysphagia, there were three categories for food and drink consistency:
- Nectar thick, the consistency of nectar, *quickly runs off* of a spoon
- Honey thick, the consistency of honey, *slowly drips off* of a spoon
- Pudding thick, the consistency of pudding, *plops off* of a spoon

Today the categories have been revised slightly to include thin, nectar-like, honey-like, and spoon-thick. These categories apply to both food and drinks.

How to Thicken Foods and Drinks
Several products are available to thicken foods and drinks. The products provide guidance on how much to add to a type of food or drink to obtain a specific consistency.

We first tried Thick and Easy, a product offered to us by the facility and made with modified food starch (usually corn, wheat, or potato based). Dad said that it took the taste out of everything. I tasted his food and drinks and I agreed. The product had the tendency to quickly overthicken and also to be lumpy. It made his drinks look cloudy. Very soon the product was causing Dad's stomach to bloat and produce gas.

After some research, we found ThickenUp which caused fewer of the problems caused by Thick and Easy. ThickenUp was made with xanthan gum instead of modified food starch. Dad said that the taste had returned to the food but his drinks were still cloudy.

In our continuing search to find a better product, we found Thickenup Clear. It was similar to ThickenUp, but it was clear and Dad's drinks were no longer cloudy.

Finally, we found SimplyThick. It came in a gel and allowed us to thicken carbonated drinks, previously not possible. Dad could again enjoy an occasional Coke.

Google "dysphagia thickeners" to find other products.

We used a little food processor to puree Dad's food with thickener. We were able to puree almost everything including meats, casseroles, pancakes and cake, and noodles could be overcooked and pureed with spaghetti sauce.

Because the thickening products had previously contained modified food starch and then xanthan gum, and they were not inexpensive nor covered by insurance, we chose to minimize their use whenever possible. We found that we could add any already thick food to get the overall thickness we desired. That included foods such as cream cheese, pudding, creamed soups and yogurt.

If we accidently overthickened food, we used water, milk, broth, gravy, tomato juice, or tomato sauce depending on what we had to thin. If we were pureeing baked ham, we added milk and cream cheese. For pureeing other types of pork, like a pork roast or tenderloin, or chicken we added broth.

Some foods did not have to be pureed. Bananas that could be mashed well, yogurt and egg salad were already appropriately thick.

Our Strategy
We had to plan, as it takes time to prepare thickened food and drinks. We also did the following.

- Dehydration is a risk with dysphagia, therefore we always had a drink by Dad's side.
  🐞🐞🐞 We always had 3-4 thickened drinks prepared in the refrigerator.

- We had go to snacks such as pudding and yogurt that did not require preparation.

- We gave Dad the same food we gave Mom, just thickened. We made sure to cook food that they liked, included foods with color and used small pretty dishes. We assured Dad that he was eating exactly what we were serving Mom, but that it just looked a little different. We created a recipe book with a section on how to prepare Dad's foods and drinks for our caregivers to use.

- We did our best to present Dad's food in as appetizing a presentation as possible. For example, we drizzled blueberry syrup on his pancakes and French toast, and gravy on his potatoes. We used spices on top of his food to add color and contrast. ***Variety, color and presentation were very important.*** *A good rule of thumb was to ask ourselves if it looked appetizing to us.* It was also important that Dad's food was served <u>as a meal</u>, giving him the opportunity *to eat different foods, instead of one food at a time or multiple foods pureed together.* It was also more appealing visually and by smell.

- We allowed plenty of time for Dad to eat. We encouraged him to swallow twice before taking another bite.

- Dad's pills had to be crushed. We had to check with a pharmacist to see what pills could be crushed and if any could be opened to put the powder into his food.

- Although Dad could brush his teeth with water, he could not swallow the unthickened water.

- Dad always had to sit up to eat, drink or take his medications.

- 👀 👀 In addition, Dad could not eat any rice unless it was in a casserole, any corn, any unthickened ice cream or any unthickened broth other than in something pureed.

Retesting

About 16 months after Dad was diagnosed, I noticed that I no longer heard any gurgling in Dad's throat and that he was not clearing it either. Dad was retested and downgraded to a honey thick consistency for drinks and allowed soft unthickened foods such as scrambled eggs or mashed potatoes. We were directed to cut meat into very small bites and mix it with mashed potatoes or something of that consistency. This made a huge increase in Dad's quality of life, as he could once again enjoy a holiday meal with a plate that looked like ours.

Ostomy Care

According to the United Ostomy Associations of America, more than 100,000 ostomy surgeries are performed every year. That number of surgeries means that at any time, between 750,000 and 1,000,000 people in the United States are living with an ostomy.

Mom needed an ostomy due to a blockage, and we didn't know anything about caring for it. The wound RN at the hospital trained my sisters and me, but we were overwhelmed and unskilled at first. The unit RNs really didn't know how to work with the ostomy, and many times it exploded all over my mom, which was not only unnecessary but also an assault on her dignity. Once Mom was home, in-home health was supposed to assist us, but they knew little more than we did about the options for supplies and the care necessary. The hospital wound RN had said to call her if we needed assistance after Mom's discharge, but she quit her job. When in-home health was no longer helping us, we were left virtually on our own. We learned almost everything through trial and error, lots and lots of errors.

It took us a long time to understand the terminology, ostomy products and the process for acquiring them. The following section is designed to provide you with the basic information needed to work with an ostomy, so that you can have a conversation with your medical professionals.

🐞🐞🐞 The United Ostomy Associations of America (UOAA) is a great resource on ostomies, ostomy products and ostomy care. UOAA's website is www.ostomy.org, and the telephone number is 800-826-0826.

What is it?
An *ostomy* is a life-saving procedure that reroutes bodily waste from its usual path in order to exit the body, usually necessary due to a blockage or a malfunction in the body's waste elimination system. The procedure creates a dark pink artificial opening, a *stoma*, on the abdominal wall through which waste material passes out of the body. A pouch is worn over the stoma to collect stool or urine. In some cases, an alternative procedure, different than a conventional ostomy, can be performed that eliminates the necessity for a pouch.

An ostomy can redirect waste from the small intestine, the large intestine or urinary tract. There are several types of ostomies.

- A *urostomy* diverts urine when the bladder has been removed or bypassed. It is sometimes confused with *nephrostomy*, which is not technically an ostomy. Instead of diverting urine out of the body through an ostomy, a nephrostomy diverts urine via a tube inserted into the bladder that drains into a pouch.
- An *ileostomy* diverts stool from the final portion of the small intestines, the ileum.
- A *colostomy* diverts stool from the colon or large intestine. It is sometimes confused with a *colonoscopy*, which is a test used to evaluate the inside of the colon.

- A *hybrid ostomy* diverts stool from the body in a location between an ileostomy and a colostomy.

A urostomy does not affect what the person can eat or drink. The exact location of the other types of ostomies within the digestive system will affect <u>what kinds of food can be eaten</u> and <u>the amount of nutrition the person will get from the food</u>.

All ostomies require careful cleaning and care to prevent skin infection.

Ostomy Products
Learning to care for Mom's ostomy was challenging at best. It required learning what options were available, and then identifying the products that would work well for Mom.

<u>Appliances</u>
While Mom was in surgery, my sisters and I were trained on ostomy care. Immediately after Mom's ostomy surgery, the wound RN tried a brand of product on Mom that did not work well. It would initially adhere to Mom's skin but minutes later would pop off. We quickly moved on to another brand. (Google "brands of ostomy supplies.")

We then had to determine whether Mom wanted to use a *one-piece or two-piece pouching system,* also called an *appliance,* which was difficult when we didn't know the pros or cons of either.

Appliances consist of two parts.
1. A *wafer, also called a skin barrier or faceplate,* serves to protect the skin around the stoma from irritation from waste. The back of it is attached with adhesive to the skin

surrounding the stoma and has a hole in the center through which the stoma is fit. The wafer also acts as an anchor for the pouch.

The wafer in either system must allow for an opening for the stoma. Some systems offer different fixed sizes of openings. Other wafers require cutting the opening to fit the stoma, which may be necessary if the shape of the stoma is irregular.

2. A *pouch*, attached or adhered to the wafer, resides on the outside of the body to collect the waste discharged from the stoma. Pouches can be transparent or opaque, drainable (open-ended, resealable) or disposable (closed-ended) and are offered in many sizes and styles. Drainable pouches are open-ended and are drained, cleaned and reused for a couple of days. Disposable pouches are closed-end pouches and are disposed of after each use.

Some pouches include a filter to allow expelled gas to escape the pouch. They include an odor-absorbent product with the filter. Whether or not the pouch has a filter, you may need to let gas out of the pouch, which can be done by opening the tail of a one-piece system or burping the wafer of a two-piece system where it snaps to the pouch. *Burping* a pouch should be done in a bathroom or private location, as fecal odor may be present.

The amount of gas produced can be affected by the person's diet. There are dietary changes necessary as a result of ostomy surgery. For example, with a hybrid ostomy, Mom had the following restrictions postsurgery: no raw celery, no skins, no casings (sausages, hotdogs), no nuts and no seeds. These foods could either clog her colon, much like a disposal gets clogged with certain foods, or would not be digested because of the location of her ostomy in the digestive tract. In addition, she continued to avoid foods that she knew made her produce gas prior to the surgery.

Appliances are either one-piece or two-piece systems.
1. One-piece appliances are manufactured with the wafer and pouch as one unit. With the one-piece system, both the wafer and pouch must be changed at the same time. With proper care, the one-piece system can be kept in place for several days.

2. A two-piece system consists of a separate wafer and pouch that are usually joined with a snap-on ring or seal. With the two-piece system, the wafer is applied to the skin and can stay there for several days. The pouch can be snapped on and left in place, or removed and emptied, cleaned or changed. While this system provides flexibility in the use of the pouch, the disadvantage is that the pouch can unexpectedly disconnect from the wafer if the seal is not properly snapped together.

🐞🐞 I experienced a pouch falling off of a two-piece appliance as I was assisting my Mom with getting onto the commode. I was standing in front of it when it literally blew off of her and it was not pleasant. The worst part was that my mom felt bad about it, and it was not her fault.

Draining the pouch
Starting immediately after surgery, you should check the pouch **every hour** to see if it needs to be emptied. Once the

patient's digestive system has returned to their normal, and you have a feeling for how often the pouch might need to be drained, you can increase the time between checks. **Always err on the side of checking the pouch too often**.

Draining the pouch is a process that takes a bit of time so be sure to set up your supplies prior to starting. It is easiest to drain the pouch while the person who wears it is on the toilet or commode. We always cleaned everything involved in the process of draining the pouch (syringe, drainage bucket) with a solution of bleach and water after each use.

🐞🐞🐞🐞 **An open-ended pouch must be drained when the pouch is ½ full**. The pouch will look like it can hold a lot more but trust me, you do not want the pouch to fill more than that before you empty it. The frequency of draining the pouch will be determined by the amount of fecal output.

🐞🐞🐞 When draining a pouch, it is important to remember to **reclose the open end**. I promise that you will only forget once. Also, clean the inside of the opening with tissue prior to closing it, otherwise the opening gets really messy.

🐞🐞🐞 Use a syringe to flush clean water into the pouch to clean it.

Changing the pouch
🐞🐞🐞🐞 **Use only water and soap** when cleaning the area around the stoma. The ingredients in many cleansing products can either cause the appliance not to adhere or cause skin irritation.

Wear time of the appliance varies. An appliance should be changed when either it has begun to leak underneath the wafer, usually indicated by odor, or it has been in use a fixed number of days. It should always be changed earlier, at the first suspicion of leakage, rather than later.

Changing the appliance involves caring for the skin and any irritations and then fitting the appliance over the stoma. It can be a very specific process, one that is based on your circumstances and the products you choose. I will not go into detail, as there are many variables, but will identify some of the additional products and accessories available to assist you.

- *Stoma paste or strip paste and adhesive rings or sprays* help to prep the skin and to improve wafer adherence to prevent leakage under the wafer. Depending on the position of the stoma, a convex ring may be needed.
- *Stoma powder* is used under the wafer to cover and protect sore skin. Stoma powder or antifungal powder can be put on in layers by applying the powder, making it damp, letting it dry and adding another layer of powder. This method is called *crusting*.
- *No-sting barrier-film spray or protector barrier wipes* help to protect the skin. We preferred the wipes.
- *Adhesive spray or liquid* can be applied to increase the adherence of the wafer to the skin.
- *Barrier rings* are used to provide additional skin protection.
- *Adhesive-removal spray or wipes* help with removing the wafer from the skin. We preferred the wipes.
- *Deodorizing drops and sprays help* to cut down on odor in the pouch. We used deodorizing drops in the pouch because they acted as a lubricant, facilitating drainage of the pouch.

- Adding *uncoated aspirin* to the pouch will help eliminate odors. We added 3-4 each time the pouch was drained. We found this to be the most effective method of eliminating odor.
- *Belts* attach to tabs on either side of the pouch, and encircle the body, lending support to the system.
- A *syringe* is used to flush the drained pouch with water to clean it.

Obtaining Supplies
Ostomy supplies are available online and at medical supply stores, and are covered by most insurance. Insurance policies usually cover a specific number of each ostomy product per month. For example, Medicare covers a fixed number of appliances per month, dependent on the type of appliance. Some supplies are covered every other month.

Some months we used more appliances than were allowed by Medicare, but we still needed them. Occasionally a scheduled delivery of supplies got delayed, putting us at risk of not having an appliance when we needed it. Therefore, we purchased additional appliances out of pocket so that we would have an emergency supply.

There were also some supplies that we preferred, barrier wipes instead of spray, that were not covered by Medicare. Therefore, we purchased those supplies out of pocket as well.

👀👀 We found the product manufacturers very helpful in assisting in fine-tuning our products, making recommendations for products and procedures as well as solving ostomy-related issues.

What Worked for Us

- Each time we changed Mom's appliance, the person doing it would date and initial the wafer with a permanent marker so that we always knew how long that appliance had been adhered to Mom and who had changed it.

- Although Mom's appliance was approved to stay on for 5 days, we changed it at least every 3 days unless it leaked sooner. We found that changing it every 3 days allowed us to prevent skin irritation and infection.

- We layered skin protection by using barrier wipes as the first layer, then stoma powder, followed by barrier spray. We then used a lot of adhesive to apply a barrier ring.

- When at home, we always had something absorbent (adult tabbed "diaper," chux, a towel) near where Mom was sitting to have it immediately available in case of an accident with her appliance. We could wrap the pouch in something absorbent and also had something there to immediately wipe up. We also did this while we were out.

- After Mom's ostomy, and because her digestive tract had been modified, she took a combination of Miralax and magnesium supplements daily.
  🐞🐞🐞 If someone is having an ostomy, they should talk with their medical provider about what might need to be added to their daily routine to maintain bowel function.

- It was critical to have a reorder schedule in place so that supplies arrived before they were needed. When a supply order arrived, we checked the inventory and restocked our supplies.

🐞🐞🐞 As I already mentioned, we had problems when Mom was in an STACH because the medical providers there did not understand the need for the additional Miralax and magnesium. They said that Mom's magnesium levels were good and that she didn't need the magnesium. They therefore told the RNs to stop giving it to Mom. My sisters and I had to advocate for Mom in order to continue the regular regimen necessary for her ostomy.

🐞🐞 Although Miralax and magnesium are generally considered safe, we had a situation after we had recently increased the amounts of these products. While at a routine doctor appointment, we found out that Mom's blood pressure was dangerously high. We took her directly to the ED, where their solution was to put Mom on blood pressure medicine. But, Mom had not previously had high blood pressure. Using our spiral notebooks, my family figured out what the problem was and lowered her dosages of Miralax and magnesium. Her blood pressure very quickly reset to its previous normal.

🐞 The procedures my family used to care for Mom's ostomy are posted on and can be downloaded from my website www.TrishLaub.com. They serve as an example only. Skin irritation and infection are concerns for those with an ostomy. We trained our in-home caregivers to care for Mom's ostomy and change her appliance. Mom had very few skin irritations, which I attribute to our procedures, standard for cleanliness and everyone's excellent care technique.

Sepsis

Mom had surgery and, only hours later, was thriving. I stayed the night and heard a change in her breathing. I checked her temperature, which had risen quickly. The medical fellow on call was in the hospital and came in to see Mom. He checked her vitals and had lab tests run with the designation "stat." There was a clear sign of an infection that had not been present prior to the surgery. She had double bladder infections, one from a nephrostomy tube and another in her other kidney. She met the criteria for severe sepsis and was rushed to the *intensive care unit (ICU)*.

The ICU doctor was supposed to have a quick family meeting, one that never happened, prior to treatment. As I walked into the room, the doctor was about to give Mom medicine via her IV. I asked about the medication and told the doctor that Mom could not have that medication. The doctor argued with me and I explained that a brief conversation with Mom's family would have identified the issue with the medicine. I demanded that the ICU doctor contact Mom's infectious disease specialist prior to administering the medication that would have had negative consequences.

While experiencing severe sepsis, Mom told my sisters and me to let her die. That was one of only two times my mom said that, so it expresses the severity of the symptoms. The decision of whether Mom lived or died was not ours to make. Our job was to ensure that she had the appropriate medical treatment for her to be comfortable and to restore quality of life for as long as possible.

What is it?
Sepsis is a life-threatening *condition* brought on by the body's response to its immune system's fight against a serious infection. Occasionally the response is negative and results in a combination of life-threatening symptoms.

How is it diagnosed?
At least two of the symptoms of sepsis must be present to be diagnosed with sepsis. The symptoms include:
- A fever above 101 degrees Fahrenheit or a temperature below 98.6 degrees Fahrenheit
- A heart rate higher than 90 beats per minute
- Respirations higher than 20 breaths per minute
- Probable or confirmed infection

Severe sepsis includes one or more of several additional symptoms such as changes in mental ability, low platelet count, problems breathing, abnormal heart functions and unconsciousness. These indicate organ failure.

Septic shock is indicated when symptoms of severe sepsis are present in addition to low blood pressure.

Blood tests and a variety of other tests are performed, depending on the symptoms.

How is it treated?
The treatment for sepsis depends on the specific cause and symptoms. Sepsis often results in admission to an ICU.

Urinary Catheterization

Mom's first medical crisis required six weeks in medical facilities. The medical providers were still working to diagnose all of her ailments, and her condition was rapidly deteriorating. Because her body was barely functioning, her bladder was not emptying. By the time anyone realized it, her bladder had 1800 ccs (500 ccs is full) of fluid in it and had almost burst. A Foley catheter was inserted to drain her bladder, and thus began the cycle of inserting a Foley, developing a urinary tract infection (UTI), removing the Foley, inserting another and developing another UTI. Of course, with each UTI Mom was prescribed antibiotics which put her at risk for C. diff. (See above.) Immediately prior to discharge, we were told that Mom would have to go home with a Foley, and would likely have to live with it forever. She did not want the Foley, because she feared that it would result in recurring UTIs and felt that eventually she would not need it. After consulting with Mom and much to the medical providers' surprise, we requested that the medical staff begin to straight catheterize Mom and to then teach my sisters and me how to do it. If we could learn to do it, we could take Mom home and work to get her to a point where she no longer needed any kind of catheterization. We learned, and within a week or two Mom no longer needed a catheter or our assistance.

What my family chose to do for our mom is not for everyone. It is a very personal procedure requiring a skill that I never thought I would have.

What is it?
Catheterization is the insertion of a hollow tube into the urethra to drain the bladder.

Why is it necessary?
Catheterization might be necessary when a person can't control when they urinate or when they have urinary retention or urinary incontinence. If urine is not emptied from the bladder, it can build up and lead to pressure in the kidneys. If too much builds up the bladder can burst.

The average bladder is designed to hold up to a maximum of 500 ccs of urine, giving the sensation of needing to be emptied when it has 250 ccs and leaving no more than 150 ccs. When I said above that Mom had 1800 ccs of urine in her bladder, which is slightly less than the contents of a two-liter bottle of pop, you can understand that it might have burst.

There are many reasons a person's bladder control can be affected, including kidney stones, inflammation as a result of surgeries and medications that impair the ability of your bladder muscles to squeeze.

Types of Urinary Catheterization
There are three main types of urinary catheters.
*   Indwelling catheters, commonly called Foley catheters, are inserted through the urethra and reside in the bladder. Occasionally they are inserted through the abdomen. These are used for both short and long term.
*   External catheters, known as condom catheters, are used primarily for men who need assistance and do not have urinary retention problems. These remain on for a day after which they are removed and reapplied.

- Short-term catheters, also known as intermittent catheters, are used for straight catheterization. The catheter is inserted and removed after the bladder empties.

All types of catheterization pose a potential for the introduction of bacteria resulting in a urinary tract infection (UTI). It is important to keep both the area where the body is entered and the catheter clean. Some catheters are for one-time use and others are reusable and require careful cleaning.

Urine collecting drainage bags should be emptied *at least* every 8 hours or as soon as the bag is full.

👀👀 Use of a squirt bottle or syringe containing a mixture of bleach and water or vinegar and water to clean the drainage bag after each draining is helpful.

My Experience with Catheterization
- I found that most facilities preferred to insert a Foley catheter as opposed to using a straight catheter. The Foley was easier for the medical professionals as, once inserted, it only required the drainage of the bag.
- Sometimes the catheter was obviously medically necessary and other times it appeared to be used for convenience when staffing was low.
- Mom had an extremely high occurrence of UTIs when Foley catheters were inserted. We never experienced a UTI as the result of using a straight catheter.
- We found that medical professionals in facilities were not skilled at straight catheterization. The procedure can be very uncomfortable if not done correctly and carefully.

- My family requested training by medical professionals in the hospital and were provided with some additional assistance from our in-home health RN. After being trained, we found that training videos on YouTube were a helpful reminder.

When using a Foley catheter, the initial objective is for a patient to be able to drain their bladder. The ultimate objective is for the person to not need the use of a catheter. The Foley, however, can cause inflammation which inhibits the bladder's ability to drain. When the medical professionals wanted to send Mom home with a Foley with the thought that she would need it forever, we had it removed and were dedicated to straight catheterizing Mom until she was able to control her bladder on her own. We started by straight catheterizing Mom every two hours, just to be sure that she was not building up urine. When we got consistent measurements that were no higher than 250 ccs, we increased the time between checks. We measured and tracked urine output and catheterized Mom three times a day until she was finally able to sense that she had to empty her bladder. The process took about two weeks, allowing the inflammation from the Foley to reduce and her bladder to return to normal function.

🐞🐞🐞 Always seek professional training on a procedure that is invasive!

🐞🐞🐞 CNAs are not licensed to do invasive procedures.

🐞

Urinary Tract Infections: UTIs

Once Mom and Dad began to require more care, they both were more susceptible to UTIs. We quickly learned to identify their symptoms. What we had been told and we quickly learned is that UTIs present differently in seniors. Once we saw the symptoms, we would call Mom's or Dad's medical professional and say that we suspected a UTI. The first question asked was always whether or not they had a fever or pain. When we said "no," we were told that there was no UTI. When we persisted and requested a urinalysis (UA,) we were correct 100% of the time. The medical providers soon learned that the changes we were observing in our parents were accurate indicators of UTIs. (See Chapter 10.)

What is it?
A UTI is an infection in the urinary tract. For those under 80, signs of a UTI are fever; frequent urination or the sensation of having to urinate; dark (dark apple juice vs lemonade), smelly (yeast-like or bad) or cloudy urine; and pain and possibly blood in the urine. *The symptoms of a UTI in those in their 80s and older are very different.* Fever and pain are not as common in those who are older, and while dark and smelly urine may occur, <u>a change in mentation is often the most obvious symptom</u>.

👀👀👀 A change in mental activity can appear as an abnormal process of thinking, such as saying something that makes no sense, and can range from slight confusion to total disorientation. If untreated, the change in mentation can quickly become as serious as the actual infection causing it.

How do you get it?
UTIs can result from any contamination with bacteria in the urethra or from urine not being flushed from the urinary system. The introduction of bacteria may be from cross-contamination from feces during cleaning after toileting. It can also result from insertion of a catheter. Another source

is from dehydration, not consuming enough liquid to cause voiding of the bladder, allowing bacteria to fester in the urinary tract.

How is it treated?
A UTI is diagnosed with a UA. Urine is collected and then tested for bacteria. Once bacteria has been identified in urine it is cultured, a process that allows the bacteria to grow in order to identify its specific strain. Upon initial diagnosis, a broad-spectrum antibiotic is often prescribed until a bacteria-specific antibiotic can be identified to match the results of the culture. Especially during the treatment of the UTI it is important to drink as much fluid as possible to flush bacteria out of the urinary tract.

What We Did to be Proactive in Identifying UTIs
UTIs are treated with antibiotics, which posed a risk of C. diff for Mom, so we were as *proactive* as possible. The sooner we identified a UTI, the sooner and more easily it could be treated.

- If there were any changes in my parents' urine output volume, we immediately began to track the volume of output and to document the color, clarity and smell of the urine.
- Mom and Dad took a supplement called D-Mannose that assists in preventing UTIs.
- We had both a toilet hat and urine cups. (See Chapter 11.) The toilet hat allowed us to capture urine and measure it using the lines on the side of the hat. The urine cups allowed us to take some of the urine for a UA.
- Once we had contacted a medical provider, we could immediately take the urine sample for testing without a parent having to leave home. Some medical providers allow for the pickup of lab samples.

Other Issues

During the time that my sisters and I oversaw the care of our parents, there were a variety of medically based issues that we had to navigate. In some cases, it was a matter of understanding who was responsible for performing a specific procedure or who would provide us with training. In others, it was determining the cause of a symptom or the need for a treatment.

A Note About Alzheimer's

My dad had Alzheimer's. I dedicated the book *A Most Meaningful Life* to detailing my experience with my dad and Alzheimer's. It starts with my initial awareness of his diagnosis and then identifies the facts and dispels the myths about Alzheimer's. Based on my family's care philosophy and our goal of providing dignified care and preserving Dad's quality of life, we developed our strategy for achieving our goal. We needed all of the information in this book, but found that when dealing with Alzheimer's there was an additional layer of care considerations necessary. That is what is identified in *A Most Meaningful Life*. My experience was that even with Alzheimer's, the possibilities are limitless and a meaningful life is possible.

A Note About Cancer

Similar to Alzheimer's, cancer has had a stigma that strikes fear in the hearts of those diagnosed and those who love them. Mom had stage 4 colon cancer that had metastasized to her liver. I will forever remember the day that I heard those words.

Years prior Mom had told me that she and Dad had decided that if they were ever diagnosed with cancer, they would not do treatment. That was based on the facts at the time that IV chemotherapy was the only treatment and it had severe side effects that diminished a person's quality of life. We learned that a lot had changed since the early days of cancer treatment, and that Mom had viable options that would not decrease her quality of life.

Mom had a colon tumor removed because it was causing a blockage. But, we were still left to deal with the cancer in her liver. For Mom, there was an oral tablet chemotherapy option. She was able to take a pill and had no negative side effects. She was also able to have a minimally invasive procedure called radioembolization, which combined embolization and radiation therapy to treat liver cancer. Both the pills and the procedure were helpful in minimizing the cancer's growth without reducing her quality of life.

Since then I have been involved with several friends who have been diagnosed with cancer, and heard about many more, who are being treated with even newer options such as proton therapy and immunotherapy. We are now seeing ads on TV for immunotherapy drugs such as Opdivo and Keytruda.

We have reached a point at which people are living quality lives with cancers that are considered noncurable. With the rapid progression of new treatments, one day soon those cancers may be curable.

Anti-clotting Medication
When a patient is in the hospital for three days or more, especially if they are having surgery or are not ambulatory, protocol is to administer anti-clotting medication. For Mom this was usually given in the form of a shot to the abdomen.

A couple of times, Mom was sent home with a prescription to continue the shots, and we were to administer them.

👀👀 In-home health professionals trained us to correctly administer the shots. It was not difficult nor painful for Mom.

Oxygen: O2
Mom had an extended stay in an LTACH and was given oxygen periodically. She had not needed oxygen prior to her stay and likely needed it due to her inactivity during her stay. At the time of discharge her oxygen was a bit low, and she was sent home with a prescription for oxygen. Once home, the oxygen arrived, and we were to keep Mom on it indefinitely, which did not make sense to us. There was no discussion about the extended need for oxygen or the option to stop using it.

At first, for a few days, we used the oxygen both day and night. Then we used the oxygen at night and worked to stop the use during the day. We initially checked Mom's oxygen level every hour. Only if it was below 90 did we use the oxygen again for an hour. When she did not need it at all during the day, we began to check her usage at night. Within a week we no longer needed to use the oxygen, but we did continue to check her oxygen on a regular basis.

There are very important safety procedures necessary when using oxygen. Please read them below.

👀👀👀 *Medical grade oxygen is highly flammable*. It is highly recommended to place an "oxygen in use" sign on the door of the home or room in which it is in use. Oxygen should be kept *at least 5 feet* from an open flame. This includes lit cigarettes, candles, fireplaces, aerosol products (air fresheners or hair spray) and flammable liquids (gasoline or lighter fluid). Research additional recommended safety procedures.

👀👀👀 If oxygen is going to be used long term in a home, it is advised to notify the gas company.

👀👀👀 The constant use of oxygen dried out Mom's nose to the point that it bled. We could use ***nonpetroleum products to moisturize her nose***.

👀👀👀 **Do not use Vaseline** to moisturize the nose of a person using oxygen because it contains petroleum. We used water-based Ky-Jelly.

👀👀 Using oxygen requires wearing a cannula, plastic tubing that hooks over your ears and goes in your nose to deliver the oxygen. The cannula wore on Mom's ears and on her cheeks. There are pads that can be put on the cannula to prevent the rubbing of the tubes on both the ears and cheeks.

Swelling of Legs

Dad's legs and feet began to swell. We began to elevate his legs during the day, but the swelling did not reduce. We were concerned that the circulation to his legs might be compromised by a blood clot or poor circulation. Reduced circulation can result in serious health risks. Although the color and temperature of his legs and feet were normal, his medical provider ordered an ultrasound to measure the blood flow through his arteries and veins. Dad's circulation was good, so we were unsure of what could be causing the problem. We then identified and evaluated any changes that had occurred in Dad's life and determined that he had unintentionally been given a higher percentage of prepared meals. These meals contained an exceptionally high level of salt, resulting in the swelling in his legs and feet. A return to his regular diet resolved the problem.

Wound Care
Mom had an abdominal infection which required wound care. In-home health professionals initially did the bandage changing but trained us on the daily care. Eventually, in-home health trained our licensed caregivers on the entire procedure.

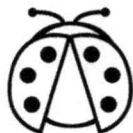

And once the storm is over you won't
remember how you made it through,
how you managed to survive.
You won't even be sure
whether the storm is really over.
But one thing is certain.
When you come out of the storm,
you won't be the same person
who walked in.
That's what the storm is all about.
Haruki Murakami

Chapter 13

FINAL THOUGHTS ...

and additional reading

It was two and a half years and the honor of a lifetime providing care for both of my parents. You have read my stories and should know that it was not easy, not because it is inherently hard, but rather I found myself lost in the darkness of the rabbit hole. I had no real experience with providing care during a medical crisis. The health care system has changed so much during my lifetime. In my constant need for answers, solutions and information, I stumbled many times, finding myself on my knees praying for the miracle of a guide to show me the way.

I have often thought that maybe my situation was so intense -- caring for both parents who were simultaneously living with multiple different conditions -- so that I would be inevitably driven to write about my experiences with the hope of helping others navigate the maze of care options and decisions.

I credit my mom for what has resulted. She was a pillar of strength and lived with more grace than I will ever have. As a child she provided me the examples of how to live and how to accept responsibility, to respond to your abilities, and do what was right, most often what was difficult. There was an unassuming beauty about Mom, one that caused strangers to stop us on the street to remark on how beautiful she was. Of course she will always be the most beautiful woman I will ever see, a beauty of which she seemed unaware. But I believe that it was not her outer beauty that drew the attention of strangers, but rather her inner beauty, her grace that shed light everywhere she went.

When I had no guide for the journey, it was her steadfast love that, like a beacon, shown light down the dark and unfamiliar path for me. How could I ever have known that I would write, in her honor, about what she facilitated? Her example motivated my unwillingness to fail at delivering the most dignified and compassionate care possible to both of my parents. Her trust and belief in me made me know that I could handle whatever came my way, that I could figure out the answers and that when no solutions were apparent, I could create one. Until her last breath, Mom facilitated the stories I have shared.

What is my mom's legacy? It is a legacy of family, helping others (especially children) whenever possible and, of course, doing the right thing, especially when it is not the easy or desired choice. Mom's is a legacy of love.

What did I take away from all that happened? I know that it is important to:

- Make good choices for your health. In spite of my dad having Alzheimer's, my parents both lived 90 years before they encountered serious health issues. My parents believed in consuming a little of everything: fruits, vegetables, meats, fish and always dessert. They were active every day and got enough sleep. They never smoked cigarettes and drank little alcohol. And as new health research became available, they adjusted their lifestyle accordingly. They lived well and still needed care, and patient advocacy, toward the end of their lives.

- Take charge of your health care. Know the options, the truth about the effectiveness and risks of medications and procedures, and make informed choices.
- Know your philosophy on medical treatment and care, as well as the end of life.
- Do the same for the ones you love who cannot care for themselves.
- Know that the real challenge is to provide dignified and compassionate care, and that in providing it, patient advocacy is the most important role.
- Remember that quality, not quantity, of life should always be the goal.

I know that I have a responsibility to care for myself and others. I have abilities and my response to them, especially in situations that are not easy or wanted, is a testament to my character. I also know that we, as a culture, have a responsibility to do better in caring for each other. We, mankind, are all in this thing called life together, and we need to take care of each other.

What if your current challenge is a call to action,
a rallying cry
that will prepare you for the next phase?
Unknown

Let my experience be your call to action! You may or may not need care someday. You may or may not be responsible for the care of another, even at their end of life. Regardless, know that the Comfort in Their Journey book series was written to guide you through the process. Unquestionably the best defense for being presented with the unknown world of care is to be prepared. The best gift you can give those you love, those who may accept the responsibility for managing or providing care for you, is presented in Chapter 2 and the Afterword of *Peaceful Endings*. Have the hard conversations about what kind of care you want and what you want for the end of your life. Have the same conversation with those you love to find out what they want. And if you are one of the projected millions whose lives will be affected by Alzheimer's, *A Most Meaningful Life* will guide you through understanding the disease, including the facts, myths and real symptoms. It identifies additional care considerations and offers limitless possibilities.

I show my scars so that
others may know they can heal.
Unknown

My mom passed away eight months after my dad. At the end of that journey, I felt battered and bloodied and emerged donning battle scars. I had fought the fight of my life to provide dignified and compassionate care, and successfully delivered the end of life both of my parents desired. The greatest toll on me was not knowing the way. It was not uncommon for me to work a care shift (anywhere from 12-36 hours awake), only to go home and spend the next 12 hours teaching myself what would be needed for questions and decisions in whatever environment in which I was overseeing their care next. Honestly, it took me a year to get back to my baseline of wellness. I do not say this to imply that your journey should or will be as challenging. I say it to allow you to understand why my hope is that my experience will spare you the same. My battle scars have healed and now are worn as a permanent sign of my love for my parents, and a reminder of my responsibility to:

- show you that even with Alzheimer's *A Most Meaningful Life* is possible

- navigate you through the maze to deliver dignified and compassionate care after you fall *Through the Rabbit Hole* and
- guide you on the walk to deliver *Peaceful Endings*

Compassion brings us to a stop,
and for a moment
we rise above ourselves.
Mason Cooley

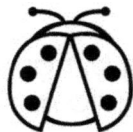

I'm a strong person
but every once in a while,
I would like someone to take my hand
and tell me
that everything's going to be all right.
Unknown

POSTSCRIPT ...

how to help someone in crisis

The first thing to understand is that a person in crisis needs help. They may not be able to ask for it. Sometimes they are too exhausted to know what they need or to even make the effort to ask for help. Everyone in a tough situation can use support. There is helpful support and misguided support. Knowing the difference makes all the difference to the one in need.

Move Love Inward, Throw The "Trash" Outward
Often at the height of a crisis, people find that they not only feel they don't know what is appropriate or helpful to say but that they in fact have said the wrong thing unintentionally.

For decades I have been aware of my relationships with others, even distinguishing between real friends and acquaintances, where real friends are let into an imaginary circle allowing them to be closer to me than acquaintances who reside in a circle further away from me. *Susan Silk, a clinical psychologist, and Barry Goldman describe a way to use that imagery to help identity what is and is not appropriate and helpful for others to say to someone in a crisis situation.* They suggest the following, which I have enhanced.

Draw a circle and write the name of the person in crisis in the center.

Draw six more circles, each larger and outside of the previous.

Label the circles, starting with the circle closest to the original, as follows

circle #2:	immediate family: significant other, children
circle #3:	close family: parents, siblings
circle #4:	true friends
circle #5:	colleagues
circle #6:	acquaintances, distant relatives
circle #7:	anyone else

The rule is simple: send your **love inward** and your ***"trash" outward.***

The person in the center can say anything, positive or negative, to anyone at any time.

For every other circle, the intention is to help those closer to the crisis, those in the smaller circles. Therefore, listening is more helpful than talking, which should provide only comfort and support. Advice should not be given to those in a smaller circle, only love and support get put in. "Trash", complaining or unhelpful personal experience or information, should be shared with bigger circles only. The trash should always be dumped out.

Most people know not to dump trash into the center ring, but many don't realize that it is never helpful to dump into any smaller circle.

Susan Silk is a clinical psychologist. Barry Goldman is an arbitrator and mediator and the author of "The Science of Settlement: Ideas for Negotiators."
OpEd piece in the LA Times 2007
http://articles.latimes.com/2013/apr/07/opinion/la-oe-0407-silk-ring-theory-20130407

What You Can Do to Help Someone in Crisis

The needs of people are variable during a time of crisis. The intensity of the crisis will ebb and flow, and with it the needs. Some crises are a sprint to a cure or a premature end and others a marathon of treatment and care. Every situation is different depending on whether the person is at home or in a facility, there are caregivers and which type, how long the crisis is likely to last and what will happen once the crisis is resolved. The person in crisis may be the caregiver (spouse, family member, friend) and/or the person needing care.

Some people will be able to provide emotional support, others logistical support and others will be organizers. If everyone uses their strengths to provide help, the person in crisis will be lifted up as much as possible.

First, ask…. "How can I help?" If you get an answer, do it. If you do not get an answer, make a suggestion, such as asking if receiving a dinner would be helpful. Sometimes people are not comfortable with accepting help, let alone asking for it. It is optimal if the person can articulate their needs. If not, sometimes it is easier for them to acknowledge whether or not a specific offer would be helpful at that time, and the offer allows them to suggest something different such as lunch instead of dinner. If you hear hesitance in their voice, you can always drop something off at their home and make it clear that you do not expect to stay and visit. If they are in need of a visit, they will invite you.

Gift cards to restaurants, in particular those offering carry out, are thoughtful. Sometimes having a gift card is the difference between whether or not the person stops to get food.

If the crisis is ongoing, you can offer to set up a calendar of food/meal deliveries, errands to be run, housecleaning etc. Ask for a list of people to contact.

Respite for the caregiver comes in many forms. If appropriate, something to brighten the person's day is nice. Think in terms of something they particularly enjoy: flowers, a sweet treat, a message, a book, or anything that will provide a moment's respite from the stress. Respite might include a visit with the person in crisis, allowing an intellectual and emotional respite for the caregiver, as well as the person being cared for, by changing the focus for a brief time. If the situation requires full-time care, a longer visit can provide the caregiver time to recharge and rejuvenate.

Whatever the method, support from friends is often what keeps someone dealing with a crisis afloat. Something as simple as a message saying that you are thinking about them can make all the difference in their day. And never underestimate the power of just listening or lending a shoulder on which to cry.

OTHER RESOURCES

Listed are few of the resources that I found most helpful. Visit www.TrishLaub.com for more resources.

The Comfort in Their Journey Book Series by Trish Laub
A Most Meaningful Life
     my dad and Alzheimer's
Peaceful Endings
     guiding the walk to the end of life and beyond
Through the Rabbit Hole
     navigating the maze of providing care

<u>Alzheimer's</u>
Alzheimer's Association
www.Alz.org
The Alzheimer's Association is an invaluable resource for anyone affected by Alzheimer's. Provides family consultation and support groups, classes, a 24-hour bilingual helpline, and safety programs that are available free of charge through individual state chapters.

Be with me Today
     A challenge to the Alzheimer's outside
By Richard Taylor, Ph.D.
DVD: HaveAGoodLife.com
A psychologist and professor diagnosed with Alzheimer's at 58 explains what it is like to have the disease, how people treat him and how they should treat him – that there is a person in there.

Contented Dementia
By Oliver James
Based on the SPECAL (Specialized Early Care for Alzheimer's) method, this book delves into the feelings and past memories that remain intact in a person living with Alzheimer's, and how both can be used to create links to the loss of more recent information.

Gates Notes, the blog of Bill Gates   www.gatesnotes.com
Why I'm digging deep into Alzheimer's blogpost

I'm Still Here
        A New Philosophy of Alzheimer's Care
By John Zeisel, Ph.D.
I'm Still Here is a guidebook to Dr. Zeisel's treatment ideas, showing the possibility and benefits of connecting with an Alzheimer's patient through their abilities that don't diminish with time, thereby offering a quality of life with connection to others.

The Spectrum of Hope,
        An Optimistic and New Approach to Alzheimer's
        Disease and Other Dementias
By Gayatri Devi, M.D.
The author defines Alzheimer's as a spectrum disease that affects different people differently. She encourages early treatment which enables doctors and caregivers to effectively manage the disease, allowing those diagnosed with it to continue to live fulfilling lives.

Dignified Care

Being Mortal
     Medicine and What Matters in the End
By Atul Gawande

In the inevitable condition of aging and death, the goals of medicine too frequently run counter to the interest of the human spirit. This book offers examples of freer, more socially fulfilling models for assisting the aging and end of life.

Honest Medicine
     Shattering the myths about aging and health care
By Donald J Dr. Murphy, M.D.

Dr. Murphy sets the record straight on popular myths, mistakes and misconceptions in regard to the controversial issues associated with health care for older patients and the importance of understanding the pros and cons of treatments.

Learning from Hannah
     Secrets for a Life Worth Living
By William H. Thomas, M.D.

Through storytelling, this book addresses the value of elders to the community as a whole and focuses on 10 principles necessary to meet their needs which include eliminating the three greatest causes of suffering: loneliness, helplessness and boredom. The 10 principles have become the basis for a real-world project, the Eden Alternative, dedicated to creating quality of life for elders and their care partners, wherever they may live.

Life After the Diagnosis
    Expert Advice on Living Well with Serious Illness
    for Patients and Caregivers
By Steven Z. Pantilat, MD
A guide to living well with serious illness and getting the best
possible end-of-life care.

End of Life

The Life Changing Magic of Tidying Up
    The Japanese art of decluttering and organizing
By Marie Kondo
This book offers a strategy for sorting through volumes of items, identifying what r what to pass along.

When Breath Becomes Air
By Paul Kalanithi
A neurosurgeon's perspective as a patient with stage 4 lung cancer and the question of what makes a life worth living.

When Souls Take Flight
    coping with grief
By Kira Rosner
A non-sectarian view of what happens when we die, with compassionate advice for anyone who is grieving.

ABOUT THE AUTHOR

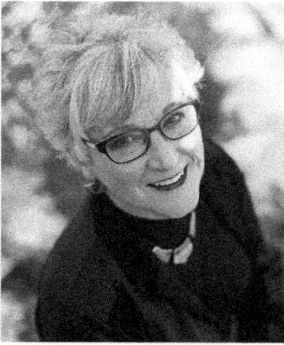

In 2002 Trish Laub was told that her father was being treated for Alzheimer's. Originally from Chicago, she and her husband moved to the Denver area in 2012 not only to enjoy the beautiful mountains but also to be closer to her parents.

Just 48 hours after Trish arrived in town, her father experienced an unexpected medical crisis, setting into motion a two and one-half year journey of care. Trish served as not only a caregiver but also as manager of both the care team and her parents' medical care. The process continued through their end of life and the settlement of their estate, and has since included the care of her mother-in-law and consulting for others. In all, over a period of five years, Trish has gained over 12,000 hours of experience in providing care for a loved one, including one living with Alzheimer's, taking the final walk of their life with them, and settling their estates.

After spending 18 years developing computer systems, Trish went on to co-found both a national dance education company and a national nonprofit prevention theater company focused on helping at-risk teens. She is a Black Belt instructor of The Nia Technique and has been licensed since 1999. Using her previous computer and teaching experience in combination with her most recent caregiving experience, Trish has created Comfort in Their Journey to provide practical guidance for dignified care through end of life.

Trish Laub
Author | Consultant | Speaker

AUTHOR
Trish is available to present her book series to your audience and to offer signed copies.

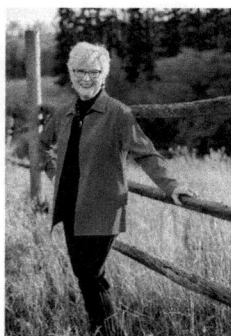

SPEAKER
Schedule Trish to bring her expertise to your group. Trish offers a variety of presentations on Alzheimer's, crisis management, end-of-life and dignified care, or can create a custom presentation for your group. She presents concise and specific information that is immediately useful, and inspires her audiences with the goal of teaching others to provide compassionate and dignified care.

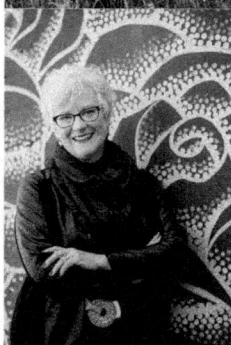

CONSULTANT
Consult Trish for guidance on meeting your caregiving needs. Trish is available to help you address your caregiving needs by discussing care options and answering your questions.

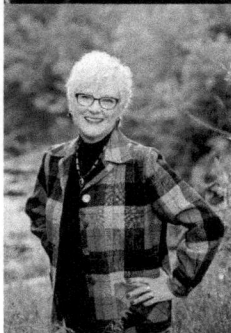

www.TrishLaub.com
720-288-0772

THE COMFORT IN THEIR JOURNEY
BOOK SERIES

A Most Meaningful Life
my dad and Alzheimer's
a guide to living with dementia

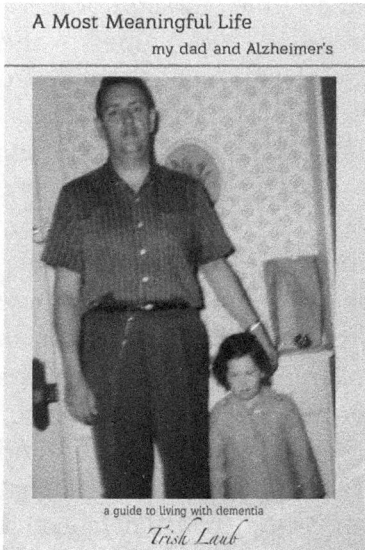

A Most Meaningful Life
my dad and Alzheimer's

a guide to living with dementia
Trish Laub

A Most Meaningful Life tells the story of a daughter's journey through Alzheimer's disease with her father, from her initial awareness of his diagnosis to navigating his care and helping him achieve the good death that we all deserve. It is the story of how Alzheimer's affected her father's life and the lives of those who loved him, as well as the story of her family's successes and failures throughout the journey. With her family's efforts, creativity and desire to preserve their father's quality of life for over a decade, he continued to truly live a meaningful life through his final days.

Through the story of her journey, the author offers a new perspective, the determination that even with Alzheimer's, the possibilities are limitless. With a clear philosophy and the creation of a strategy, others can have a roadmap to navigate their loved one's journey so that they have "A Most Meaningful Life."

Peaceful Endings
guiding the walk to the end of life and beyond
steps to take before and after

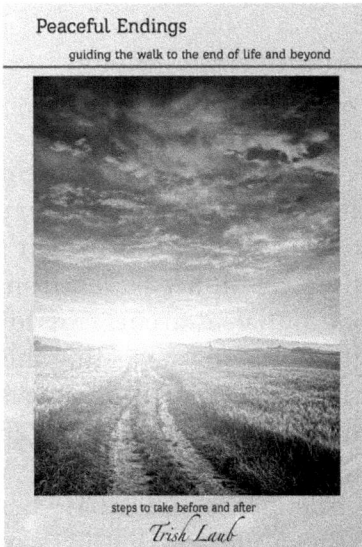

Peaceful Endings

guiding the walk to the end of life and beyond

steps to take before and after

Trish Laub

The topic "no one wants to talk about," end of life and beyond, is exactly what *Peaceful Endings* addresses. Many times the end of life is preceded by illness and caregiving, and may also include a variety of crises, as life changes and decisions must be made quickly. Whether proactively preparing for the end of life, or facing it imminently, there are medical, legal, financial, insurance and care decisions to be made, each with its own specific language. The author walks the reader through the terminology, the choices and the process of the end of life. The author also details what must be done after the transition, and provides perspective on stepping into a new normal after a loved one's life has ended.

Through the Rabbit Hole
navigating the maze of providing care
a quick guide to care options and decisions

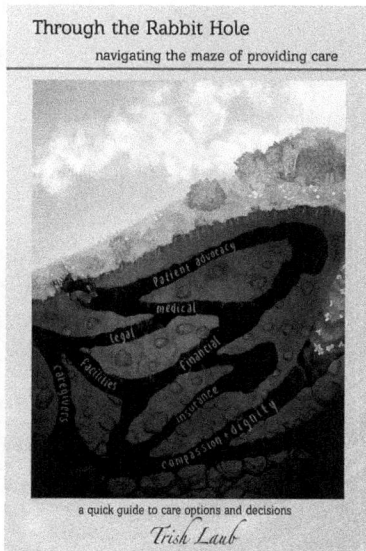

Through the Rabbit Hole is exactly the reference book that the author needed for quick access to information during her experience providing care for her ill parents. It wasn't available for her, so she has written it for all the families and caregivers who are now beginning their journeys. Her parents' medical crises caused her to fall down the rabbit hole and into the maze of unfamiliar options and decisions. Having emerged from the maze, the author details the complexities of caregivers and facilities, the need for patient advocacy, as well as the medical, legal, financial and insurance aspects of care. With the end goal of compassionate and dignified care, this book, a wonderful companion to *A Most Meaningful Life*, is a beacon through the maze of care.

288

Comfort in their Journey
with Trish Laub

Whether during an illness or injury, or at the end of life, I hope that you have found your purchase helpful in your journey of providing compassionate and dignified care.

VISIT THE COMFORT IN THEIR JOURNEY WEBSITE
Go to www.TrishLaub.com to check out everything Trish has to offer including a blog containing new information and topics not covered in the book series.

While you are there… please send us a review to post.

COMING IN SPRING 2019
The CitJClub membership including access to the information in all three books in the series, including search capabilities across all three books, and much more.

Your purchase of this book qualifies you for a discounted CitJClub membership.
Visit www.TrishLaub.com for more information.
720-288-0772

www.ingramcontent.com/pod-product-compliance
Lightning Source LLC
Chambersburg PA
CBHW070910030426
42336CB00014BA/2351